MUSCLEGATE:
THE NEW SCIENCE OF GAINING MUSCLE FASTER

AN ESSENTIAL GUIDE FOR COACHES, PERSONAL TRAINERS, AND BODYBUILDERS

MANUAL GONZALEZ

Musclegate: The New Science Of Gaining Muscle Faster

© 2022 Manual Gonzalez

ISBN 978-1-66782-951-7

eBook ISBN 978-1-66782-952-4

CONTENTS

CHAPTER 3: INTENSITY OF
EFFORT DURING EACH SET 52

CHAPTER 5: THE OPTIMAL NUMBER OF SETS FOR MUSCLE GROWTH................. 96

CHAPTER 6: REPETITION SPEED & NUMBER OF REPETITIONS FOR OPTIMAL MUSCLE GROWTH......... 127

INTRODUCTION

The Watergate scandal was one of the biggest political scandals of the early 1970s. This political cover-up led to the resignation of Richard Nixon, but the – *gate* scandal did not end there. The Merriam-Webster dictionary defines the use of the suffix – *gate*, "referring to a scandal or a cover-up." The – gate scandals have been ongoing, such as *Irangate, Bridgegate, Climategate*, and the most recent sports-related scandal, *Spygate* and *Deflategate*. Hundreds of new exercises are posted on social media and fitness websites every day, claiming these exercises build muscle faster than traditional exercise. As a result of the misinformation and social media spreading articles and videos with no scientific credibility at an unprecedented rate, many athletes and fitness enthusiasts can lose months or even years of progress following a resistance training program. The *MuscleGate* scandal of exercises that promise to build muscle faster is growing at an exceedingly rapid rate. For example, a traditional standing biceps curl is not enough to grow bigger biceps with today's social media. I once saw a guy on Instagram *standing on one leg* doing a bicep curl, stating that it was more effective than traditional biceps curls. Based on what research is this coming from?

People believe that if an exercise is harder to perform, it must be better! Another workout trend for getting better results is balance board training. Balance board training involves performing an exercise on an unstable surface, which proponents claim results in greater muscle activation and greater increases in muscle mass. One study found a decrease in force production by 60% in exercises in the bench press when performed on a stability ball.[1] Performing exercises on a stability ball can diminish the tension placed on the muscle, leading to a subpar increase in muscle growth. Instability exercises emphasize core strength. They can be used for general fitness and may be helpful during periods of recovery and recuperation. Still, instability ball training is inferior to traditional resistance exercise for increasing strength or muscle mass.[2] Instability ball training is not recommended for hypertrophy (i.e., muscle growth) or strength training because it does not provide a sufficient stimulus to induce muscle growth. Muscle growth is the process of progressively increasing muscle tension.

Social media influencers and major news outlets have a major impact on people exercising and buying sports nutrition supplements. Each week, articles are posted about how Hollywood actors got in shape for their roles in the movies, such as "How Chris Hemsworth Got Ripped to Play Thor." This has led to the mentality to copy celebrities' routines on social media to build muscle. This often leads to a body dysmorphia of regular gym-goers into an unrealistic expectation of how they should look. A recent study of regular gym participants found a negative relationship between comparing others' physiques on social media and their own body image. This led to greater body dissatisfaction and the use of dietary supplements (i.e., protein, creatine, pre-workouts, etc.) and anabolic steroid use. The study found that 65% of the participants use the internet, and 32% use social media as their primary source of information on dietary supplements.[3]

---

1 Kenneth G. Anderson and David G. Behm, "Maintenance of EMG Activity and Loss of Force Output with Instability," *Journal of Strength and Conditioning Research* 18, no. 3 (August 2004): 637–40.

2 Ronald Snarr et al., "Instability Training: Help or Hype?," *Personal Training Quarterly* 2 (March 1, 2015): 4–8.

3 Luuk Hilkens et al., "Social Media, Body Image and Resistance Training: Creating the Perfect 'Me' with Dietary Supplements, Anabolic Steroids and SARM's," *Sports Medicine – Open* 7, no. 1 (November 10, 2021): 81.

There are hundreds of exercise programs that claim to build muscle faster. This has led to mass confusion about the best way to build muscle. Should I use short rest periods? Should I train with more or fewer sets? This has led to "program jumping." A person is jumping to the newest workout fad every week to gain muscle. One week its SuperSets, then its high-intensity training, and then its high-volume training. It's overwhelming to find the right answer. It's not uncommon to see fitness magazines on the grocery store counter with titles such as *"Gain an Inch on Your Biceps in Four-weeks!"* and *"Build a Chest like The Rock!"* leading to unrealistic expectations about how much muscle you can gain from a program.

Some people are still doing fasted cardio in the morning to burn more body fat, based on a book that is a decade old. A 2017 study of the literature found no evidence of fasted cardio for reducing body fat or changes in body fat.[4] Meaningful weight loss and fat loss are achieved by caloric restriction, not fasted cardio. The title MUSCLEGATE is a term I find perfect for the fitness industry because there is so much misinformation and scandals about building muscle. Please take a moment to think of the millions of dollars made from such fitness products with zero science to support their claims, such as the Shake Weight, Thighmaster, Vibro-Belt, The Slim Suit, and the Body Blade. There is a multi-million-dollar industry for females wearing waist slimmer's (i.e., an elastic compression that compresses the abdomen) to give an hourglass figure. Not only are these not effective, but they can also weaken abdominal muscles, compress internal organs, reduce blood flow (i.e., blood flow decreased to fingertips by ~36%), and lead to reduce breathing.[5,6]

---

4 Daniel Hackett and Amanda D. Hagstrom, "Effect of Overnight Fasted Exercise on Weight Loss and Body Composition: A Systematic Review and Meta-Analysis," *Journal of Functional Morphology and Kinesiology* 2, no. 4 (December 2017): 43.

5 Youngjoo Na, "Clothing Pressure and Physiological Responses According to Boning Type of Non-Stretchable Corsets," *Fibers and Polymers* 16, no. 2 (February 1, 2015): 471–78.

6 Terrence Green and Amanda Roby, "The Effect of Waist Trainers on Breathing," *Respiratory Care* 63, no. Suppl 10 (October 1, 2018).

THE MUSCLE GROWTH VORTEX OF CONFUSION

If you think about the amount of misinformation in the fitness industry, it is staggering! Here is a shortlist of things advocated to get in shape faster:

- Don't want to diet? You can get shredded abs with the six-pack abs stimulator in which you stick electrodes on your stomach and have the machine stimulate the muscles to contract. Unfortunately, despite these products still being sold today, they don't work!

- A 2005 study found that 12 weeks of abdominal stimulation (i.e., ab contracting device) in track and field athletes found no changes in abdominal oblique muscles or subcutaneous fat thickness in the ab-stimulating groups or control groups after the intervention period.[7]

- The dumbbell pullover in which you lie on a bench has been advocated as a chest exercise to "stretch the ribcage" and give a lifter a bigger chest. Today, we know that the dumbbell pullover is a poor activator of the chest muscles compared to the bench press. The dumbbell and barbell pullover results in greater activation of the lats and triceps and cannot be recommended as a complementary exercise for the chest.[8]

---

7 Taku Wakahara and Ayumu Shiraogawa, "Effects of Neuromuscular Electrical Stimulation Training on Muscle Size in Collegiate Track and Field Athletes," *PLOS ONE* 14, no. 11 (November 13, 2019): e0224881.

8 Yuri de Almeida Costa Campos and Sandro Fernandes da Silva, "Comparison of Electromyographic Activity during the *Bench Press* and *Barbell Pullover* Exercises," *Motriz: Revista de Educação Física* 20 (June 2014): 200–205.

- Many people will often imply that because an exercise has greater muscle "activation," it leads to greater muscle growth. Using muscle activation cannot be used to imply greater muscle growth.[9] A perfect example of this is hamstring activation increases during a squat (i.e., 30.24%). However, yet little muscle growth of the hamstrings occurs during squats.[10]

The list goes on and on for exercises that were once thought to build muscle but have now been debunked.

THE "MEATHEAD" YEARS

A "meathead" is described in the *Urban Dictionary* as *"An enormously muscular guy who cannot hold a conversation about anything other than weightlifting and protein shakes."* Yes, I considered myself a 'meathead' since I was a teenager and picked up my first bodybuilding magazine. Sadly, I was not an enormously muscular guy, but my life revolved around protein shakes, bodybuilding magazines, and the latest exercise routine to build muscle. I would read the bodybuilding magazines each month to learn the latest exercise techniques to build muscle. I tried to mimic the routines of great bodybuilders such as Arnold Schwarzenegger. I tried Supersets, Drop Sets, 100 rep set, German Volume Training, SuperSlow, Muscle Confusion, Giant Sets, Instinctive Training, adding more sets, changing reps, training more frequently, eccentric exercise, and just about any other new training principle that promised more muscle growth. I jumped from program to program, trying to find the "secret program" that all the jacked bodybuilders were using. I would pick up *FLEX* and *Muscle and Fitness;* each magazine

---

9 Andrew D. Vigotsky et al., "Greater Electromyographic Responses Do Not Imply Greater Motor Unit Recruitment and 'Hypertrophic Potential' Cannot Be Inferred," *Journal of Strength and Conditioning Research* 31, no. 1 (January 2017): e1–4.

10 Keitaro Kubo, Toshihiro Ikebukuro, and Hideaki Yata, "Effects of Squat Training with Different Depths on Lower Limb Muscle Volumes," *European Journal of Applied Physiology* 119, no. 9 (September 2019): 1933–42.

article had some huge guy screaming in pain, with some insane weight that they were using. Based on what I read every month, you had to train your ass off and annihilate every muscle group if you wanted to gain muscle. I believed the pros used some "secret" training system to get results. They were bigger than everyone else because they were training harder.

My training was not enough based on my poor results, so I started using all the latest muscle-building supplements in the magazines and spent thousands of dollars on these ingredients, now debunked by science. Some of the embarrassing things I did to attempt to gain muscle were:

- Drinking 5000 calorie mass-building shakes.

- Training twice a day because I read that exercise-induced increases in anabolic hormones produced during exercise were the key to muscle growth.

- Performing 100 rep squats to shock muscles into growth.

- Getting up in the middle of the night to drink a protein shake to stay "anabolic."

- Placed electrodes on various body parts to stimulate muscle growth.

- I read a book that recommended that one should squat three times a week and drink a gallon of whole milk every day to gain more muscle.

Chances are, you have probably done some of these things to build muscle as well. Science has debunked all these concepts. It's embarrassing everything I did to build muscle, so hopefully, you can save your money and train more intelligently than I did with the concepts outlined in this book.

In hindsight, I realized I wasn't building muscle, not because I was not consuming enough calories or because I was not training hard enough. I had no structure in my training routine. I went to the gym religiously and thought I just needed to lift heavy weights. I had no plan, never kept a training journal to measure training volume (i.e., sets x reps x weight), and never took a deload (i.e., a structured rest period) to recover. Don't expect impressive gains in muscle if you don't have a plan. I did not understand the fundamentals of training periodization and emphasized supplements rather than a well-balanced diet. I just followed the routines in the magazines and thought that gaining muscle just meant to train harder and use more weight. The key to building more muscle is not found in the popular fitness magazines or an Instagram celebrity's newest workout, training technique, or supplement. The best place for accurate information on the latest muscle-building research is Pubmed (i.e., database of science and biomedical topics in the science journals). You can build an imposing physique based on science-driven information rather than relying on fitness magazines, Instagram celebrities, and supplement hype. The muscle biologists on Instagram and Twitter that promote their new research findings on muscle growth don't have millions of followers like the jacked social media stars; unfortunately, most of the studies they publish go unnoticed. This book will debunk all the fitness myths and give you the tools to build more muscle in less time, based on the work of the leading scientific experts in muscle physiology.

THE REAL SUPERHEROS

Before we get into the biggest myths generated by the fitness industry to gain more muscle, it's important first to give credit to the authentic heroes. Over the past two decades, there has been an enormous increase in articles regarding protein synthesis, protein breakdown, and muscle growth. A special thanks to all the Ph.D.'s, muscle biochemists, exercise physiologists, and others that have written research articles, applied for grants, and conducted endless hours to conduct and publish these studies. They are the staunch champions of this book. This book would not be possible if I did not credit all the academics involved in muscle biology research, which is the foundation of this book. Every research study required hundreds of grueling hours of data collection, statistical analysis, and was published in a peer-reviewed journal. Their hard work has resulted in many training philosophies once thought of as the foundation of building muscle is now debunked!

NO MAGIC PROGRAM WORKS FOR EVERYONE

I would love to say that I have a "secret" training program included in this book that guarantees that you build muscle; unfortunately, I don't. There is no workout program, but it has the research behind the fundamentals of growing muscle. No one program will work for everyone. This book aims to help you understand what the current research recommends to build muscle faster and change your routine to best fit your needs. *Every resistance exercise program needs to be individualized to each person's genetic potential for recovery.* The inter-individual variation in genetics for the improvements in components of aerobic exercise, strength, and power can be explained by genetics up to 44, 72, and 10%, respectively.[11] Therefore, following a person's exercise program will often not work for two different people because of a strong genetic component for influencing results. There are basic principles from the research that you can use as a starting point, but no magic program works for everyone. I leave the exercise selection, sets, reps, rest period, and training techniques for you to decide. If you are looking for a thorough analysis into the physiology of muscle growth, please refer to such books as *Science and Development of Muscle Hypertrophy* and *NSCA's Essentials of Sport Science.* I have tried to keep this book as simple as possible without getting into too much detail about complex muscle physiology. This book focuses on the research behind the popular training techniques advocated to boost muscle growth faster, such as training to failure, rest period duration, repetitions in reserve, exercise

---

11 Henry C. Chung et al., "Do Exercise-Associated Genes Explain Phenotypic Variance in the Three Components of Fitness? A Systematic Review & Meta-Analysis," *PLOS ONE* 16, no. 10 (October 14, 2021): e0249501.

intensity, volume, eccentric overload, drop sets, supersets, etc. Each chapter covers the most popular gym myth regarding building muscle and *actual* research studies using the training principle.

The Chapters are broken down into short sections. The book has a popular fitness myth about building muscle, **MUSCLEGATE**. The correct answer is then given **THE TRUTH EXPOSED. WALK OF SHAME** are some of the most embarrassing things that I have done in my past to gain more muscle!

EXAMPLE:

MUSCLEGATE: FOLLOW THE BIGGEST GUY IN THE GYM ROUTINE TO BUILD MUSCLE

THE TRUTH EXPOSED: The most jacked guys will post their latest workout routine on social media and get millions of views. If it works for them, it must work for you. Most of the biggest guys in the gym are genetically gifted and can gain muscle quickly. They may also use massive amounts of performance-enhancing drugs or have extremely gifted genetics, or a combination of both. Some people are known as what researchers refer to as *hyper-responders* or extreme responders. These people grow like crazy in response to resistance exercise.[12] They are genetically gifted to grow muscle faster compared to others.

Contrary to genetically gifted people, some people are known as hard gainers or low-responders; for some reason, these people don't gain muscle easily because of genetic differences. For example, in one training study, low responders had either no change or a pathetic ~4% increase in muscle growth. In contrast, high responders experienced a 30% increase in muscle

---

12 Michael D Roberts et al., "Physiological Differences Between Low Versus High Skeletal Muscle Hypertrophic Responders to Resistance Exercise Training: Current Perspectives and Future Research Directions," *Frontiers in Physiology* 9 (July 4, 2018): 834–834.

growth, despite using the same routine.[13] The research also suggests that high responders lose more muscle mass after detraining (i.e., stop training) than low responders. After detraining, high responders lost 10.5% muscle mass, whereas low responders only lost .6% muscle mass.[14] So, high responders gain muscle faster, but they also lose muscle faster when they stop training. Some studies have found that the range of muscle growth can vary between – 2% gains to a 59% increase in muscle growth and strength gains between 0 to +250%. A study of 585 subjects who followed the same training program looked at the differences in muscle growth responses:

- 232 subjects gained increases in muscle size between 15-25%,

- 10 subjects gained 40%, and

- 36 subjects gained less than 5%.[15]

This suggests that everyone gains muscle at a different rate to a resistance training protocol. What works for one person may not work for another. Just because someone has a poor response to an exercise protocol does not mean they are doomed. It just means they have not found the correct training protocol that best fits their genetics. The traditional advice given to those that don't grow muscle easily or hard gainers is to do fewer sets and take more rest days; however, this is contrary to what research finds (Chapter 5). Hardgainers may simply need to increase the number of sets or increase training frequency. As you will read later, some people have better muscle growth when they increase their sets, whereas others make better gains when they decrease their sets!

---

13 M. V. Franchi et al., "Muscle Thickness Correlates to Muscle Cross-Sectional Area in the Assessment of Strength Training-Induced Hypertrophy," *Scandinavian Journal of Medicine & Science in Sports* 28, no. 3 (March 2018): 846–53.

14 Aapo Räntilä et al., ~High Responders to Hypertrophic Strength Training Also Tend to Lose More Muscle Mass and Strength During Detraining Than Low Responders,~ *The Journal of Strength & Conditioning Research* 35, no. 6 (June 2021): 1500–1511.

15 Monica Hubal et al., "Variability in Muscle Size and Strength Gain after Unilateral Resistance Training," *Medicine and Science in Sports and Exercise* 37 (June 1, 2005): 964–72.

MUSCLE GROWTH IS AN INDIVIDUAL PROCESS

Just because someone looks great and uses a particular protocol does not mean it will work for you. Today, many people will follow an Instagram celebrity and follow the exact workout thinking; if it works for them, it will work for me. This mentality is not a scientific approach to gaining muscle. Unless the workout plan is from an identical twin, chances are what works for someone else won't necessarily work for you. Treat your body as an experiment and try different training techniques to see what works best for you.

The key to muscle growth is to track your progress. Keeping a training journal, getting body composition regularly assessed, monitoring your psychological state (i.e., Do you feel motivated to go to the gym?), monitoring your physiological symptoms (i.e., Are you feeling fatigued during exercise?), and making sure your diet is meeting caloric needs to support your training are all important for tracking your progress.

CHAPTER 1:

RESEARCH

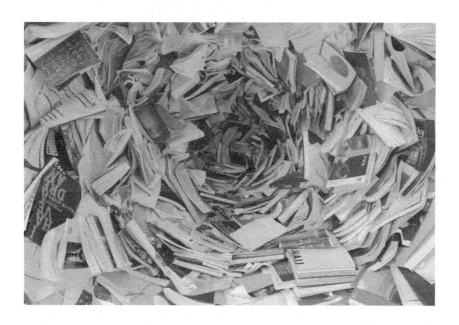

RESEARCH STUDIES: AN EPIC CLUSTERF&%K

Before beginning this journey of debunking some of the greatest myths based on training and muscle growth, it's important to understand the issues regarding the research process. A single research study is more like a piece of a gigantic puzzle; it gives us a clue of the big picture. *Never assume that a single study gives you a definitive answer.* When I first started on this journey of using peer-reviewed research studies to determine what's true and what's bogus for causing muscle growth, one of the first studies that I looked at was SuperSlow Training (i.e., lifting and lowering the weight at a very slow speed). One study found that SuperSlow training resulted in better muscle gains than traditional training, and I thought I had discovered the secret training principle to unlock muscle growth. As you will later read in Chapter 6, SuperSlow is not the greatest training principle to gain muscle…in fact; it sucks! I took *one study* result with untrained subjects and jumped to the conclusion that this *one study* was the definitive missing link to muscle growth. I was completely misguided in using one study to say that a training principle is the *Holy Grail* of training. Muscle growth occurs as a principle of muscle overload! As you will learn later, many studies have shown that traditional training is better for increasing lean mass than SuperSlow.[16] SuperSlow may work well for beginners; however, those with training experience will benefit from traditional resistance exercise for gaining lean muscle mass.[17] Other issues in research studies comparing the effects of two different resistance exercise protocols for muscle growth are that the sets or total workload for two workouts are different so that one group is doing more exercise. The subjects did not gain muscle because they used some magic training principle. They grew more muscle because they were doing more exercise, which resulted in greater tension on the muscle. When studies are designed to make sure that both groups are doing the same amount of total workload (sets x reps), the results in muscle growth are many times similar.

A similar occurrence can occur in protein supplementation studies, in which one group consumes a protein supplement after exercise gains more muscle. Was it because the group consuming the protein supplement after exercise caused more muscle growth? It could be that the protein supplement group consumed more total protein per day than the control or experimental group, which resulted in greater muscle growth. Total protein intake is a better predictor of muscle hypertrophy than the

---

16 Laura K. Keeler et al., "Early-Phase Adaptations of Traditional-Speed vs. Superslow Resistance Training on Strength and Aerobic Capacity in Sedentary Individuals," *The Journal of Strength & Conditioning Research* 15, no. 3 (August 2001): 309–14.

17 Amichai Lyons and James R. Bagley, "Can Resistance Training at Slow Versus Traditional Repetition Speeds Induce Comparable Hypertrophic and Strength Gains?," *Strength & Conditioning Journal* 42, no. 5 (October 2020): 48–56.

timing of protein.[18] Total protein intake comprising a complete spectrum of essential amino acids is more important than the protein source.[19] A 2019 meta-analysis found that protein supplementation above 1.6 g/kg/bw (.7 grams per pound of body weight) provided no further increases in lean muscle mass.[20] However, later studies have suggested that more protein is needed on training days (i.e., 2.0 g/kg/bw or 1 gram per pound of body weight) to maximize the anabolic response to resistance exercise.[21] The International Society of Sports Nutrition recommends for building muscle mass, an overall protein intake of 1.4-2.0 grams per kg of body weight per day (i.e., .6-1 gram per pound of body weight) and for fat loss, higher protein intake at 3.0 g/kg/day (i.e., 1.4 grams per pound of body weight).[22] Thus, it is recommended that at least 1 gram of protein per pound of body weight be consumed on training days.

Always remember that one study never proves a training principle works! It certainly adds new knowledge to the scientific literature, but never base your training beliefs on a single study. The same holds true for any new supplement studies that are released.

---

18 Brad Jon Schoenfeld, Alan Albert Aragon, and James W. Krieger, "The Effect of Protein Timing on Muscle Strength and Hypertrophy: A Meta-Analysis," *Journal of the International Society of Sports Nutrition* 10, no. 1 (December 3, 2013): 53.

19 Victoria Hevia-Larraín et al., ~High-Protein Plant-Based Diet Versus a Protein-Matched Omnivorous Diet to Support Resistance Training Adaptations: A Comparison Between Habitual Vegans and Omnivores,~ *Sports Medicine (Auckland, N.Z.)* 51, no. 6 (June 2021): 1317–30.

20 Robert W. Morton et al., "A Systematic Review, Meta-Analysis and Meta-Regression of the Effect of Protein Supplementation on Resistance Training-Induced Gains in Muscle Mass and Strength in Healthy Adults," *British Journal of Sports Medicine* 52, no. 6 (March 1, 2018): 376–84.

21 Michael Mazzulla et al., "Protein Intake to Maximize Whole-Body Anabolism during Postexercise Recovery in Resistance-Trained Men with High Habitual Intakes Is Severalfold Greater than the Current Recommended Dietary Allowance," *The Journal of Nutrition* 150, no. 3 (March 1, 2020): 505–11.

22 Ralf Jäger et al., ~International Society of Sports Nutrition Position Stand: Protein and Exercise,~ *Journal of the International Society of Sports Nutrition* 14, no. 1 (June 20, 2017): 20.

THE NEWEST SUPPLEMENT
MUSCLE GROWTH CRAZE

A decade ago, when chromium picolinate supplements first came out, every bodybuilder and lifter bought this hot new supplement because *one* new research study showed that it could increase muscle mass and strength in football players. Unfortunately, no one checked the study, and some red flags influenced the study results. The football players taking chromium picolinate were likely *chromium deficient* because of excessive sweating and nutritional deficiencies. If you are chromium deficient, then yes, adding this essential mineral back to your diet will increase muscle growth; however, most people that are not chromium deficient do not have the same effects on muscle growth.[23] This is an example of taking a single study and extrapolating the results to the general population.

Another example is the testosterone-boosting supplement D-Aspartic acid. A preliminary investigation found that D-Aspartic acid boosted testosterone in men with low testosterone. This led to a surge in sales in D-Aspartic acid supplements in resistance-trained men hoping to boost testosterone. When researchers administered D-Aspartic acid to healthy young men with normal testosterone, there was no change in testosterone or lean muscle mass compared to a placebo.[24,25] Even worse, high dosages of D-Aspartic acid resulted in a decrease in testosterone.[26] These are just a

---

23 P. M. Clarkson, "Effects of Exercise on Chromium Levels. Is Supplementation Required?," *Sports Medicine (Auckland, N.Z.)* 23, no. 6 (June 1997): 341–49.

24 Blair Crewther et al., "Short-Term d-Aspartic Acid Supplementation Does Not Affect Serum Biomarkers Associated With the Hypothalamic–Pituitary–Gonadal Axis in Male Climbers," *International Journal of Sport Nutrition and Exercise Metabolism* 29, no. 3 (May 1, 2019): 259–64.

25 Geoffrey W. Melville, Jason C. Siegler, and Paul W. M. Marshall, "The Effects of D-Aspartic Acid Supplementation in Resistance-Trained Men over a Three Month Training Period: A Randomised Controlled Trial," *PloS One* 12, no. 8 (2017): e0182630.

26 Geoffrey W. Melville, Jason C. Siegler, and Paul Wm Marshall, "Three and Six Grams Supplementation of D-Aspartic Acid in Resistance Trained Men," *Journal of the International Society of Sports Nutrition* 12 (2015): 15.

shortlist of supplements with preliminary positive results that generated millions of dollars in supplement hype that failed to meet expectations.

FACTORS INFLUENCING RESEARCH RESULTS

When looking at a training principal effect on muscle growth, it's best to look at a meta-analysis (i.e., collection of studies and analyzing the results). This is an extensive collection of data points, and researchers are better able to compare the results of many studies instead of just one study. The beauty of a meta-analysis is that it analyzes many studies with conflicting results, which results in a greater statistical power due to the greater number of subjects, greater diversity of subjects, etc., resulting in a greater confirmation of the data analysis. When analyzing a research study, many factors can affect the study's outcome. Some factors are:

- Training status of a subject (i.e., trained vs. untrained)

- Age (i.e., young vs. elderly adults)

- Genetics (i.e., a hyper-responder can affect the mean outcome of the study)

- Exercise selection (multi-joint vs. single-joint exercises)

- Were the subjects consuming the same macronutrients (Protein, fat, and carbohydrates)?

- Were the sets taken to complete muscular failure or not?

- How did they assess body composition? (i.e., DEXA, BIA, MRI, etc.)

- The sample size of the study (i.e., how many subjects)

- Were the total training loads equated in the study (i.e., was one group doing more than the other?)?

- Training adherence (i.e., were the training groups supervised in a laboratory, or were they unsupervised and told to perform the program on their own)

- Type of statistics used to analyze the results

- Duration of the study

- Lifestyle factors (i.e., sleep, life stress, etc.)

- Author bias (Does the lead author have a vested interest in the study's outcome?)

Any of these variables can affect the outcome of the study. One of the biggest learning lessons was that just because a particular training design reached statistical significance does not mean it translates into real-world results. Many factors can affect the outcome of a study, and human studies are difficult to control. Human test subjects are notorious for not correctly reporting things regarding self-reporting data, especially regarding diet. For example, a college student is in a resistance training study determining the effect of a particular training principle, but he is sleeping 4-6 hours a night, eating twice a day, and drinking alcohol and not reporting it. What do you think the outcome of the results will be? The outcomes of using college students are hard to extrapolate to serious athletes and bodybuilders eating 4-6 meals a day, sleeping 8 hours a night, and adhering to a well-designed periodized resistance training protocol.

RATTED OUT RESEARCH STUDIES

The beauty of using rats and other animals in a research study is that you can control what they eat, their training, when they sleep, etc. One of the biggest mistakes I have made reading animal research is extrapolating the results to humans. Animal studies are a great exploratory way of looking at muscle growth, but the research does not always translate into real-world results. For example, some of the first animal studies on placing a muscle in a stretched position resulted in large increases in muscle growth. However, it's entirely unrealistic to think that similar results can apply to humans. For example, one bird study found that stretching a muscle resulted in a 318% increase in muscle growth. However, the bird's muscle was put in a stretched position for *28 days*.[27] Don't think stretching your muscle for 2 minutes will translate into a 318% increase in muscle growth! Just because it works in rats or mice, don't conclude that it can work in humans. Believe it or not, researchers can make rats squat and increase leg muscle growth![28] They take a rat and make it wear a vest attached to a wooden arm that can have weights added to it weekly, mimicking a progressive overload resistance training protocol. All we need now is to get another rat to spot him!

SELF-REPORTED DATA...LIAR...LIAR

In research data collection with humans, controlling all the factors affecting the outcome of a study is more challenging. Researchers do their best to ensure that the group's behavior and lifestyle are tightly regulated. Self-reported data is notorious for being wrong. The classic study was that women claimed they were "small eaters," and they could not lose weight, no matter what they ate. The women were placed on a diet. The researchers used doubly labeled water (i.e., the gold standard for measuring energy expenditure) and compared this to their food journals. Their food reported journal intake of the women who claimed they could not lose weight was 1,340 calories, but their actual calorie intake from doubly labeled water was 2,586 calories. When the women were supplied their meals from the laboratory and told only to eat the food provided to them, they lost 1.65 pounds

27 J. Antonio and W. J. Gonyea, "Progressive Stretch Overload of Skeletal Muscle Results in Hypertrophy before Hyperplasia," *Journal of Applied Physiology (Bethesda, Md.: 1985)* 75, no. 3 (September 1993): 1263–71.

28 T. Tamaki, S. Uchiyama, and S. Nakano, "A Weight-Lifting Exercise Model for Inducing Hypertrophy in the Hindlimb Muscles of Rats," *Medicine and Science in Sports and Exercise* 24, no. 8 (August 1992): 881–86.

per week.[29] This shows that human self-reported data is often wrong, and human data collection is often under-reported or over-reported.

BE OBJECTIVE WHEN READING RESEARCH

In one of the first sports science conferences that I attended, I grasped how many variables can affect the outcome of a study. It amazed me when a researcher presented his study findings only at the end would other leading researchers in the same field point out research flaws in the study design that could have affected the study results. It's like a Twitter battle in a presentation room, and the arguments can get quite heated! When one researcher presents conflicting data compared to what has been previously established by others, it can be a royal rumble!

I have learned a valuable lesson that one study does not mean it's the definitive answer. It's not uncommon for an investigation to find positive results, and another study will test the same variables and find negative or contradictory results. *I can guarantee that in every study I point out in this book, you can find opposite studies that contradict it.* In this book, there are many instances where results show beneficial findings in one study and contradictory studies regarding the same exercise principle. Unfortunately, this is the research process for muscle growth; there is no simple answer. The key to reading research is to be objective. Now that we have gone over all the things that can go wrong when reading a research study, let's get into the practical applications of the research findings and leave the statistical analyses to the feuding professors. When looking at a research study, always look at the *training status* of the subject to make realistic comparisons.

---

29 D. Clark et al., "Energy Metabolism in Free-Living, 'Large-Eating' and 'Small-Eating' Women: Studies Using 2H2(18)O," *The British Journal of Nutrition* 72, no. 1 (July 1994): 21–31.

MUSCLEGATE: THE TRAINING STATE OF THE SUBJECT DOES NOT MATTER

THE TRUTH EXPOSED: The training state of the subjects enrolled in the study has a major outcome on muscle growth results. *Untrained subjects or people who have never lifted weights* will make greater gains in strength and muscle growth than well-trained athletes. Untrained subjects, or what the industry calls *newbies,* make unbelievable gains in strength and muscle size when exercising. When untrained athletes first begin weight training, the first few weeks of resistance training result in large increases in strength, mainly increased through neurological adaptations (the nervous system learns a new movement), while gains after that are primarily because of increases in muscle.[30,31] It's kind of like watching a new baby learn to walk because he is trying to teach his nervous system to coordinate with his muscles to move. The same process takes place when you are starting to lift weights. You are teaching your body an entirely new movement pattern in which it must learn. Remember when you first started working out, your strength seemed to skyrocket? Well, that's because your nervous system is adapting and enhancing neural pathways to your muscles. The nervous system can increase muscle strength in response to resistance exercise by increasing the speed of the impulse or strength of the impulse.[32] Strength increases result from your nervous system being able to perform an exercise movement better.

It's not uncommon for untrained subjects to achieve as much as 40% strength gains. *However, trained and elite trained athletes can make strength*

---

30 Michael R. Deschenes and William J. Kraemer, "Performance and Physiologic Adaptations to Resistance Training.," *American Journal of Physical Medicine & Rehabilitation* 81, no. 11 Suppl (November 2002): S3-16.

31 T. Moritani and H. A. deVries, "Neural Factors versus Hypertrophy in the Time Course of Muscle Strength Gain," *American Journal of Physical Medicine* 58, no. 3 (June 1979): 115–30.

32 Per Aagaard et al., "Increased Rate of Force Development and Neural Drive of Human Skeletal Muscle Following Resistance Training," *Journal of Applied Physiology (Bethesda, Md.: 1985)* 93, no. 4 (October 2002): 1318–26.

gains of ~16% and 2%, respectively.[33] Untrained subjects' muscles grow quickly due to starting a new program. This is commonly called *Newbie Gains*. Untrained athletes have greater increases in muscle protein synthesis, whereas trained athletes have a dampened effect (discussed in Chapter 2). For trained athletes, it's much more challenging to gain muscle. There is a "ceiling effect" for trained athletes; they reach the upper limit of muscle growth in part mainly due to genetics and a dampened anabolic response to resistance exercise, so gaining muscle is much more challenging. Most of the people reading this book, I assume, would have several years of training. So, before you read a study and think it applies to you, make sure the subjects are *resistance-trained* with several years of resistance exercise experience in the methods section to make realistic comparisons. I wish I could say that every study in this book used resistance-trained men and women with five years of training, eating 1.5 grams of protein per pound of body weight, and doing everything possible to gain muscle. Unfortunately, I can't say that. Many university studies use recreational college lifters, and getting the subjects enrolled in a study is difficult. You have to get Institutional Review Board approval and other things that are a complete nightmare for researchers.

WALK OF SHAME: I read an exciting research study in a fitness magazine showing that the subjects using this new supplement gained twice the increase in muscle mass compared to those not taking the supplement. I ran to GNC and bought the product and didn't see any gains in muscle like the study. This was most likely because I had been training for several years and increasing muscle mass is much harder for more advanced athletes. Supplement companies love to use untrained subjects in their studies because their strength and muscle gains are larger than those of well-trained. For example, a 21-week training study found that untrained

---

33 Thomas R Baechle, Roger W Earle, and National Strength & Conditioning Association (U.S.), *Essentials of Strength Training and Conditioning* (Champaign, IL: Human Kinetics, 2008).

subjects had significant increases in strength (20.9%) and muscle growth (5.6%). In contrast, strength-trained athletes increased maximal force of 3.9% and no changes in muscle cross-sectional area (-1.8%).[34] If you are looking at a supplement study, make sure the participants in the study *are well-trained* with several years of experience.

CHAPTER SUMMARY:

- Many different variables can affect the outcome of muscle growth in a study.

- Most studies will use untrained subjects (i.e., college students) who respond differently than trained individuals.

- It's not uncommon to see one study find a particular exercise technique that increases muscle growth, and the following month, a study will contradict these findings.

- A meta-analysis is the best way to look at training techniques because it collects many studies.

- Trained athletes will have a much harder time increasing muscle growth because there is a "ceiling effect" they are reaching.

---

34 Juha P. Ahtiainen et al., "Muscle Hypertrophy, Hormonal Adaptations and Strength Development during Strength Training in Strength-Trained and Untrained Men," *European Journal of Applied Physiology* 89, no. 6 (August 1, 2003): 555–63.

CHAPTER 2:

FACTORS FOR BUILDING MORE MUSCLE

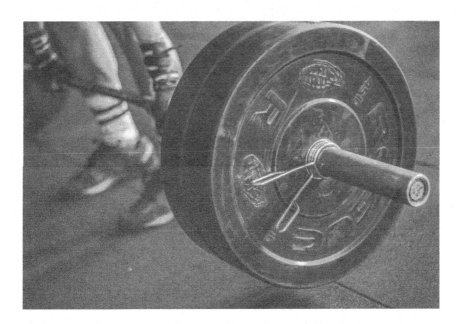

WORKOUT ADHERENCE:
THE MOST IMPORTANT TRAINING VARIABLE

Before we get into the different mechanisms of muscle growth, I will start with the one principle that is more important than any other training principle: workout adherence. If a person can't stick to a training program, all the advanced training techniques won't matter if they can't adhere to a regimented training program. There must be consistency in a program to achieve results. If a routine is unmotivating to perform, don't expect consistent gains in strength and muscle mass. Some programs advocated to build muscle, such as the 5 X 5 program, are so monotonous, they have a low program adherence because of lack of variety. The 5 X 5 program advocates greater strength and muscle mass and involves performing heavy weights with five sets of five reps, with compound movements such as squats, bench press, and deadlifts. The downsides of the 5 X 5 program are that there lacks variety in rep ranges (i.e., 10-20 repetitions) with higher rep ranges, and consistently using heavier weight can add extra stress to the joints and ligaments. A program that advocates increasing muscle mass at the increased risk of injury is a double-edged sword for lifters. There is certainly nothing wrong with a program like this, and it may be beneficial to incorporate it into your routine for a strength cycle phase. However, it probably won't work for people in the long term who want a variety of exercises in their workout.

A suitable muscle growth training protocol motivates the client to keep using the program. Find exercises that you truly enjoy doing to make the most progress. If you hate doing squats, don't do them! Don't perform exercises that cause joint pain or movement discomfort! There are plenty of other exercise alternatives that can build muscle. For decades, it was preached that you need to perform bench press to build a big chest. Many of the top bodybuilders do not perform bench press, but they do many other exercises to stimulate chest growth. If your biceps hurt due to tendonitis or other joint issues while doing barbell preacher curls, try cable preacher curls. They are equally effective for increasing muscle growth.[35] Never think that one exercise has to be performed to increase muscle size; there are always alternatives.

---

35 João Pedro Nunes et al., ~Placing Greater Torque at Shorter or Longer Muscle Lengths? Effects of Cable vs. Barbell Preacher Curl Training on Muscular Strength and Hypertrophy in Young Adults,~ *International Journal of Environmental Research and Public Health* 17, no. 16 (January 2020): 5859.

MUSCLEGATE: HIIT IS THE ONLY WAY TO LOSE BODY FAT

THE TRUTH EXPOSED: HIIT or high-intensity interval training has been growing in popularity due to its purpose of getting in and out of the gym faster, with better results. HIIT exercise modalities encourage the individual to "exercise as hard as you can." Some people like high-intensity workouts, whereas others will not. Some people have intensity-preference traits that influence how a person feels during exercise.[36] If you are a personal trainer, starting a client off with a high-intensity exercise may not be the best approach for client adherence. At lactate threshold, or the point at which lactate starts to increase, is where workout displeasure rises. There is large variability when this point occurs in many people. *Exercise intensity that is self-selected rather than imposed results in greater tolerance to higher exercise intensity.*[37] It has been found that some people love high-intensity, whereas others prefer a more moderate-intensity exercise. If you are a personal trainer, your goal is to help your clients gain muscle by sticking to a program that works best for them. Not all clients will start at the same workout intensity; the key is to develop an individual program that fits each person's needs. Most importantly, a program that results in a high adherence level. If a person views high-intensity exercise as unpleasant, this will likely result in low long-term adherence. Despite the numerous benefits of high-intensity training, the physiological benefits that can be

---

36 Allyson G. Box and Steven J. Petruzzello, "Why Do They Do It? Differences in High-Intensity Exercise-Affect between Those with Higher and Lower Intensity Preference and Tolerance," *Psychology of Sport and Exercise* 47 (March 1, 2020): 101521.

37 Panteleimon Ekkekakis, Gaynor Parfitt, and Steven J. Petruzzello, "The Pleasure and Displeasure People Feel When They Exercise at Different Intensities: Decennial Update and Progress towards a Tripartite Rationale for Exercise Intensity Prescription," *Sports Medicine (Auckland, N.Z.)* 41, no. 8 (August 1, 2011): 641–71.

gained from high-intensity training will be meaningless if a person can't adhere to the program.[38]

For decades, it has been emphasized that HIIT training is superior for fat loss to moderate-intensity exercise. A recent meta-analysis found that both moderate-intensity cardio and interval training resulted in similar reductions in body fat as well as changes in lean mass.[39] The author concluded, "Our findings provide compelling evidence that the pattern of intensity of effort and volume during endurance exercise [i.e., interval training vs. continuous training] has minimal influence on longitudinal changes in fat mass and fat-free mass, which are likely to be minimal anyway." Find a program that best fits your client's intrinsic exercise motivation needs. Find out a person's goals starting a training program and guide them towards realistic expectations. It's been found that from a targeted list of 21 possible reasons for weight training, three motives were ranked the highest: personal challenge, physique anxiety, and mood control.[40]

THE KING OF MUSCLE GROWTH: TENSION

The primary mechanism in which muscles grow is *tension*.[41] In the late 60s researcher Alfred Goldberg, a Harvard Professor of Cell Biology, had an interest in muscle growth and protein synthesis and breakdown. In experiments with rats, he quickly realized that their muscles grew rapidly due to

---

38 Allyson G. Box and Steven J. Petruzzello, "High-Intensity Interval Exercise: Methodological Considerations for Behavior Promotion From an Affective Perspective," *Frontiers in Psychology* 12 (2021): 41.

39 James Steele et al., "Slow and Steady, or Hard and Fast? A Systematic Review and Meta-Analysis of Studies Comparing Body Composition Changes between Interval Training and Moderate Intensity Continuous Training," *Sports (Basel, Switzerland)* 9, no. 11 (November 18, 2021): 155.

40 NEIM N. EMINI and MALCOLM J. BOND, "Motivational and Psychological Correlates of Bodybuilding Dependence," *Journal of Behavioral Addictions* 3, no. 3 (September 2014): 182–88.

41 Brad J. Schoenfeld, "The Mechanisms of Muscle Hypertrophy and Their Application to Resistance Training," *Journal of Strength and Conditioning Research* 24, no. 10 (October 2010): 2857–72,

tension overload. Tension is such a powerful promoter of muscle growth that they could do many things to see if they could blunt muscle growth from occurring. They removed the rat's pituitary so they could not produce Growth Hormone (GH) and Insulin-Like Growth Factor-1 (i.e., IGF-1 invokes potent anabolic action in muscle), castrated them so they could not produce testosterone, removed their thyroid, or just didn't feed them… despite this punishment, the rats still had increases in muscle growth when tension was applied to the muscle.[42] In his research, Dr. Goldberg stated,

"Maximal tension development leads to increases in muscle hypertrophy. Unlike normal developmental growth, work-induced hypertrophy can be induced in hypophysectomized (rats that can't produce GH) or diabetic animals (produce no insulin—an anabolic hormone). This process, thus, appears independent of growth hormone and insulin, as well as testosterone and thyroid hormones. Hypertrophy can also be induced in fasting animals, in which there is generalized muscle wasting. Thus, muscular activity takes precedence over endocrine influences on muscle size."

Besides tension, muscle stretch is a potent stimulus for muscle growth. Animal studies in which a muscle is placed on chronic stretch results in muscle growth. Stretching a muscle with tension overload results in more muscle growth than tension overload alone. For example, in a review of the animal studies that looked at mechanisms of muscle growth:

- Stretching + tension overload=20.95% increase in muscle growth.
- Exercise alone=11.59% increase in muscle growth.

The author concluded that "It appears that hyperplasia (increases in muscle cell fiber number) muscle cell in animals is greatest when certain types of mechanical overload, particularly stretch, are applied."[43] Whether

---

42 Alfred L. Goldberg et al., "Mechanism of Work-Induced Hypertrophy of Skeletal Muscle," *Medicine and Science in Sports and Exercise* 7, no. 4 (1975): 248.

43 George Kelley, "Mechanical Overload and Skeletal Muscle Fiber Hyperplasia: A Meta-Analysis," *Journal of Applied Physiology* 81, no. 4 (October 1, 1996): 1584–88.

hyperplasia occurs in humans is an intense debate, but the two principles that have been shown to enhance muscle growth in humans are tension and muscle stretch. Combining these two principles results in two specific increases in muscle growth. *Tension overload increases the muscle's size, whereas stretching muscle results in an increase in the muscle's length.*[44] To emphasize the importance of how a combination of tension overload and stretching a muscle influences the growth of muscle fascicle length (i.e., each fascicle is a bundle of muscle fibers), twenty-eight men were divided into various groups and took part in a 10-week leg strength-training program twice per week. The traditional strength group used the same external load for both eccentric and concentric phases throughout the program, whereas another group was assigned to an accentuated eccentric loading group. The accentuated eccentric loading group performed strength training with an additional load during the eccentric phase of each repetition (+ 40% greater than the concentric phase). The accentuated eccentric loading group combined two powerful stimuli: tension overload with stretch. Despite both groups using the same training volume, only the accentuated eccentric loading group showed significant increases in fascicle length after the training period (vastus lateralis: ~14% increase, vastus medialis: ~19% increase). These findings suggest that higher load eccentric training evokes greater fascicle length increases than lower load concentric training.[45] Other contributing factors that may contribute to greater gains in muscle mass from accentuated eccentric loading are increased androgen receptors, IGF-1, and several myogenic regulatory factors (myoD, myogenin,

---

44 Kent W. Jorgenson, Stuart M. Phillips, and Troy A. Hornberger, "Identifying the Structural Adaptations That Drive the Mechanical Load-Induced Growth of Skeletal Muscle: A Scoping Review," *Cells* 9, no. 7 (July 2020): 1658.

45 Simon Walker et al., "Increased Fascicle Length but Not Patellar Tendon Stiffness after Accentuated Eccentric-Load Strength Training in Already-Trained Men," *European Journal of Applied Physiology* 120, no. 11 (November 1, 2020): 2371–82.

MYF5, MRF4, HGF, and myostatin).[46] This re-emphasizes the importance of tension overload for maximal increases in muscle hypertrophy.

FACTORS INFLUENCING MUSCLE GROWTH

Resistance exercise leads to a cascade of events that increase muscle protein synthesis. Several training variables have been found to impact muscle growth:

- High muscular tension (training with sufficiently heavy weight).

- Sufficient time exposure to that tension (training with enough sets/reps and/or frequencies).

- Sufficient effort (sets should be performed close to the proximity of muscular failure).

- Range of Motion (training at stretched muscle length)

To maximize muscle growth, you need a combination of all four. Other variables contributing to muscle growth are metabolic stress and muscle damage, but these are debatable.[47] Metabolic stress and muscle damage *may* contribute to muscle growth, but muscle tension is the king. You may wonder how big a factor tension is for muscle growth; well, if you ever had a cast on for several weeks, you would see how fast a muscle will atrophy. No tension equals no muscle growth. If you go from an active lifestyle to a sedentary lifestyle, muscle loss occurs. Researchers found that if a healthy subject went from an active lifestyle of 13,054 steps per day to a sedentary lifestyle of 1,192 steps, the loss of activity resulted in decreased protein synthesis by 27% and an increase in the muscle suppressing hormone

---

46 John P. Wagle et al., "Accentuated Eccentric Loading for Training and Performance: A Review," *Sports Medicine* 47, no. 12 (December 2017): 2473–95.

47 Henning Wackerhage et al., "Stimuli and Sensors That Initiate Skeletal Muscle Hypertrophy Following Resistance Exercise," *Journal of Applied Physiology (Bethesda, Md. : 1985)* 126, no. 1 (January 1, 2019): 30–43.

myostatin.[48] Muscle disuse results in "anabolic resistance," accompanied by reductions in muscle protein synthesis. This means the anabolic action in muscle are suppressed. As little as 2 weeks of reduced walking results in reduced protein synthesis, with rates declining ~13–26% from baseline.[49] For building muscle, "USE IT OR LOSE IT!"

MUSCLE FIBER TYPES

Human skeletal muscle is predominantly composed of three types of muscle fibers: Type I fibers, Type IIX, and Type IIA.

Type I fibers are also known as slow-twitch fibers. Type I fibers have high aerobic capacity and are better suited for muscle endurance training, such as endurance competitors like marathoners and triathletes. Type I fibers are characterized by low force/power/speed production, high endurance, and fatigue resistant. Type I fibers have the least potential for muscle growth. There is evidence of fiber-type transitions that occur with specific training modalities. Researchers investigated the effects of 13 weeks of marathon training on fiber type shifts in novice runners. Leg muscle Type I fiber composition increased by 8%, suggesting muscle fiber transitions to a more aerobic-based capacity with specific training modalities.[50]

Type IIX fibers are characterized by high force/power/speed production and low endurance. Type IIX are called fast-twitch fibers and have a greater capacity for muscle growth. The fiber profile of Type IIX shifts towards Type IIA fibers when people use bodybuilding protocols and other anaerobic based exercises such as sprinting. When weightlifting, Type IIX,

48 Brandon J. Shad et al., "One Week of Step Reduction Lowers Myofibrillar Protein Synthesis Rates in Young Men," *Medicine and Science in Sports and Exercise* 51, no. 10 (October 2019): 2125–34.

49 Leigh Breen et al., "Two Weeks of Reduced Activity Decreases Leg Lean Mass and Induces 'Anabolic Resistance' of Myofibrillar Protein Synthesis in Healthy Elderly," *The Journal of Clinical Endocrinology and Metabolism* 98, no. 6 (June 2013): 2604–12.

50 N. Luden et al., "Skeletal Muscle Plasticity with Marathon Training in Novice Runners," *Scandinavian Journal of Medicine & Science in Sports* 22, no. 5 (2012): 662–70.

fast-twitch fibers drive explosive power when doing 1RM or sets of low, heavy repetitions. A study in subjects trained with fast, explosive isokinetic resistance training for ten weeks found a decrease in Type I fibers (53.8% to 39.1%), with a simultaneous increase in the percentage of type IIX fibers (5.8 to 12.9%).[51]

Type IIA fibers are a combination of Type I and Type IIX fibers; they are a hybrid of both. They have a fast contraction velocity and are more resistant to fatigue than Type IIX. Type IIA are most often increased during bodybuilding style routines and other anaerobic sports that involve a high anaerobic capacity. It's been found that 8 weeks of sprint training increased the proportion of Type IIA fibers (from 31.2% to 46.8%) in the legs, with a corresponding reduction in the percentage of Type I fibers (from 50% to 43%) and Type IIX fibers (18.8% to 10.5%).[52]

---

51 D. Paddon-Jones et al., "Adaptation to Chronic Eccentric Exercise in Humans: The Influence of Contraction Velocity," *European Journal of Applied Physiology* 85, no. 5 (September 2001): 466–71.

52 J. L. Andersen, H. Klitgaard, and B. Saltin, "Myosin Heavy Chain Isoforms in Single Fibres from m. Vastus Lateralis of Sprinters: Influence of Training," *Acta Physiologica Scandinavica* 151, no. 2 (1994): 135–42.

Characteristics of the 3 Muscle Fiber Types

Muscle Fiber Comparison

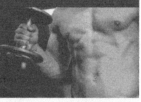

Characteristics	SLOW TWITCH TYPE I	FAST TWITCH TYPE IIA	FAST TWITCH TYPE IIX
Contraction Time	Slow	Fast	Very Fast
Aerobic Capacity	High	Moderate	Low
Diameter	Small	Medium	Large
Resistance to fatigue	High	Moderate	Low
Force Generating Capacity	Low	Moderate	Very High
Fibers per Motor Unit	<300	>300	>300
Capillaries per Fiber	High	Moderate	Low
Creatine Phosphate	Low	High	Highest
Anaerobic Capacity	Low	High	Highest

THE TYPES OF CONTRACTIONS THAT CAN INFLUENCE MUSCLE GROWTH

Repetitions are further broken down into three components: a concentric phase (lifting the weight), isometric phase (muscle is contracting, but no joint movement is occurring), and an eccentric phase (lowering the weight). If you were using the leg extension, the lift would begin with a concentric phase in which the weight is lifted. The isometric phase is when the weight is paused at the middle of the movement, and finally, an eccentric phase when the weight is lowered.

Contracting (concentric) and stretching (eccentric) muscles are crucial for muscle growth. Contrary to belief, isometric training (no movement) can increase muscle growth.[53] Isometric exercise places tension on the muscle, but the active contracting and stretching of muscle results in superior muscle growth. It's not uncommon to see people in the gym lifting a weight with no control; however, it's important to understand that tension and also the tension duration on the muscle is much more important than the weight. This means that a maximal lift lasting a few seconds will be inferior to muscle growth using a lower weight, but more tension on a muscle over a longer time. Researchers found that when subjects trained with 75% of a maximal voluntary contraction, sustained muscle contractions in the leg extension (contracted the legs explosively for 1 sec, but held the contraction for 3 seconds) resulted in more than a 3-fold greater increase in muscle growth than explosive contractions (contracting as hard and as fast as possible).[54] *This shows that muscle growth depends not only on the weight but also on loading duration (i.e., time).* This simple study is a good analogy for muscle growth responses between powerlifting and

---

53 Dustin J. Oranchuk et al., "Isometric Training and Long-Term Adaptations: Effects of Muscle Length, Intensity, and Intent: A Systematic Review," *Scandinavian Journal of Medicine & Science in Sports* 29, no. 4 (April 2019): 484–503.

54 Thomas G. Balshaw et al., "Training-Specific Functional, Neural, and Hypertrophic Adaptations to Explosive vs. Sustained-Contraction Strength Training," *Journal of Applied Physiology (Bethesda, Md.: 1985)* 120, no. 11 (June 1, 2016): 1364–73.

bodybuilding protocols. Powerlifting protocols use peak tension for a short time frame, whereas bodybuilding protocols result in greater sustained tension for a more prolonged period.

Isometric exercise places tension on the muscle, but no active stretch will result in lesser muscle growth than actively contracting the muscle.[55] By actively stretching and contracting the muscle, you expose different muscle fibers to a wide variety of external stressors. *As mentioned previously, each contraction (i.e., concentric and eccentric) causes a different type of muscle growth.* Hence, both are equally important. One study found that lifters who did not pause (i.e., eliminated the isometric contraction pause between contractions) between concentric and eccentric contractions had similar increases in muscle growth to those who paused for one second in the isometric position between contractions.[56] This is not to say that isometric contractions are unnecessary, just of lesser importance than concentric and eccentric contractions for muscle growth.

TENSION AND ALSO *TIME* IS IMPORTANT FOR MUSCLE GROWTH

If you compare the muscle size of bodybuilders to pure strength athletes, there is a noticeable muscle size difference. Bodybuilders train with less weight but use more sets and reps, resulting in more tension on the muscle over time, whereas powerlifters train with very heavy weight, which results in greater peak tension but less total tension over time. The biggest misconception among lifters is that *only heavy weight can increase muscle growth.* If heavy weights were the best way to generate muscle growth, doing maximal weights with singles and doubles would produce maximum muscle

---

55 Rodrigo Vanerson Passos Neves et al., "Dynamic, Not Isometric Resistance Training Improves Muscle Inflammation, Oxidative Stress and Hypertrophy in Rats," *Frontiers in Physiology* 10 (January 22, 2019): 4.

56 Michiya Tanimoto and Naokata Ishii, "Effects of Low-Intensity Resistance Exercise with Slow Movement and Tonic Force Generation on Muscular Function in Young Men," *Journal of Applied Physiology (Bethesda, Md.: 1985)* 100, no. 4 (April 2006): 1150–57.

growth, but this is not the best way because the tension on the muscle is very brief because of the low number of reps. The tension must be of sufficient duration and progressively increased over time to stimulate muscle growth. It's well documented that increasing volume (i.e., total workload) is especially important for advanced lifters to increase muscle growth, whether by adding more weight or more sets/reps.

SUMMARY

- Muscle fibers can increase in size (diameter) or increase in length.

- High muscular tension, sufficient time exposure to that tension,

- and sufficient effort is required for muscle growth.

- Repetitions should be completed through a full range of motion.

Several bodybuilding magazines have talked about the importance of continuous tension for greater muscle growth. One of the most common principles that trainers use is to ensure that their athletes never lockout at the end of a set to keep continuous tension on the muscle. For example, if you are doing triceps extensions, you would not fully lock out the elbows at the end of the movement, because this will reduce tension on the muscle. It's suggested that more tension is placed on the muscle by not locking out on exercise movements, and more muscle growth occurs.

MUSCLEGATE: NEVER LOCKOUT AT THE END OF A REP

THE TRUTH EXPOSED: You will accumulate more fatigue and metabolic stress if you don't "lock out" at the end of the repetition. Metabolic stress was once considered a major mechanism of muscle growth, but lately, the research seems to suggest it may not be as important as researchers once thought it was. One study found that subjects who lifted a weight in 1 second and lowered in 1 second with no pause with a heavier weight (i.e.,~80% 1RM) training to complete failure had similar increases in muscle growth as those who exercised with a lighter weight (~50% 1RM) with a slow lifter speed and a 1 second pause (3 seconds concentric, 3 seconds eccentric, 1 second isometric) training to failure.[57] Despite having similar increases in muscle hypertrophy, the group that eliminated the isometric contraction (i.e., no pause) had greater metabolic stress consisting of higher lactate and lower muscular oxygenation. Another study by the same research group had subjects train with either constant tension (i.e., no pausing at the end of a repetition) or a regular resistance exercise group. Both groups trained to failure with the same exercises: machine squat, chest press, lat pulldown, abdominal crunch, and back extension. The normal group performed each exercise with a full range of motion, using an 80–90% one-rep max load and a 1-second lifting, 1-second lowering, and 1-second pause phase. The constant-tension group avoided locking out the joints, so there was continuous tension. They used a 55–60% one-rep max load and a 3-second lifting and 3-second lowering phase; there was no pause phase. *At the end of the study, both groups increased muscle mass similarly.* This suggests that whether you want to lockout at the end of a repetition or keep continuous tension with no lockouts are both capable of increasing muscle growth if you train to failure.[58] One important note, the continuous tension group used much less weight (i.e., 55-60% of a 1RM) but still built the same amount of muscle as the heavier weight group (i.e., 80-90% of a 1RM). This points to the fact that using a lighter weight until muscular failure with no lockouts at the end of a repetition can build similar muscle growth as a heavier weight with a lockout. This again points to

---

57 Tanimoto, M., & Ishii, N. (2006). Effects of low-intensity resistance exercise with slow movement and tonic force generation on muscular function in young men. Journal of applied physiology (Bethesda, Md. : 1985), 100(4), 1150–1157.

58 Michiya Tanimoto et al., "Effects of Whole-Body Low-Intensity Resistance Training with Slow Movement and Tonic Force Generation on Muscular Size and Strength in Young Men," *Journal of Strength and Conditioning Research* 22, no. 6 (November 2008): 1926–38.

using lighter weights for periods to give tendons and ligaments recuperation time from using heavier weight while not sacrificing muscle.

BLOOD FLOW RESTRICTION TRAINING

Blood flow restriction (BFR) utilizes a tourniquet or other compression device around a muscle to reduce blood flow and create metabolic stress. It has been suggested that metabolic stress stimulates muscle growth. Does this mean you should start using BFR training to increase muscle size? If you look at the research, BFR training and moderately heavy weight programs (>65% of a 1-RM) result in similar increases in muscle growth.[59] BFR training can be good for injured people or people in rehabilitation because it incorporates very light weights but increases muscle growth. Some studies have found heavy lifting to have a slight edge in increased muscle and strength compared to whole-body BFR training.[60] If you want to experiment with BFR training, it may be worth trying on stubborn body parts that you are having issues growing, such as the calves and arms.[61] It has been documented that blood flow restriction training can result in similar increases in muscle growth as a high-rep, light weight traditional resistance training program, despite a lower training volume.[62] A 2021 study found that calf muscle thickness was increased after blood flow restriction training in well-trained resistance exercise men, despite using a lower training

59 Manoel E. Lixandrão et al., ~Magnitude of Muscle Strength and Mass Adaptations Between High-Load Resistance Training Versus Low-Load Resistance Training Associated with Blood-Flow Restriction: A Systematic Review and Meta-Analysis,~ *Sports Medicine (Auckland, N.Z.)* 48, no. 2 (February 2018): 361–78.

60 Brandner, C. R., Clarkson, M. J., Kidgell, D. J., & Warmington, S. A. (2019). Muscular Adaptations to Whole Body Blood Flow Restriction Training and Detraining. Frontiers in physiology, 10, 1099.

61 Joshua Slysz, Jack Stultz, and Jamie F. Burr, "The Efficacy of Blood Flow Restricted Exercise: A Systematic Review & Meta-Analysis," *Journal of Science and Medicine in Sport* 19, no. 8 (August 2016): 669–75.

62 Christopher A. Fahs et al., "Muscular Adaptations to Fatiguing Exercise with and without Blood Flow Restriction," *Clinical Physiology and Functional Imaging* 35, no. 3 (May 2015): 167–76.

volume. In the study, resistance-trained men exercised with 4 sets at 30% 1-RM until failure with and without a BFR cuff placed below the knee. At the end of the study, the average number of repetitions completed per training session across was higher in the no BFR group compared (i.e., 70 reps) to the BFR group (i.e., 52 reps). Despite the higher training volume, the traditional resistance training group had slightly less muscle growth (+1.94%) than the BFR group (3.29%).

You can mimic BFR training or metabolic stress training without occluding blood flow. Researchers had subjects do BFR training with leg extension (20% of a 1-RM) in which they occluded blood flow with a cuff, or they had subjects do a leg extension but held their legs in the extended position (isometric position) for 5 seconds and squeezed as hard as they could with 20% of a 1-RM. At the end of the study, both groups had similar increases in leg size.[63] BFR training induces metabolic stress and less muscle damage than traditional exercise. Still, it has been found to induce similar or slightly less muscle growth than traditional resistance exercise.

If constant tension caused by not locking out and creating metabolic stress was the key to muscle growth, then BFR training with continuous blood flow restriction should result in more muscle growth than BFR than with breaks or removing the BFR between sets. Researchers assigned participants to a BFR group (wore restrictive cuffs during and between sets) or a BFR group in which they removed the BFR (deflated for 30 seconds between sets). At the end of the study, both groups of BFR training, whether they left the cuffs on the entire workout or removed them between sets, equally increased muscle growth. Interestingly, despite more metabolic stress with the BFR cuffs left on for the entire workout period, similar increases in muscle growth occurred when participants were allowed to remove the BFR cuffs between sets. Pain levels and effort were higher in

---

63 Carolina Brandt Meister et al., "Effects of Two Programs of Metabolic Resistance Training on Strength and Hypertrophy," *Fisioterapia Em Movimento* 29 (March 2016): 147–58.

the BFR group that left the cuff on the entire workout.[64] This study suggests that more metabolic stress will not always result in more muscle growth. I think this is a perfect analogy to not locking out the joints to keep continuous tension and create more metabolic stress. No further increases will be beneficial once a certain metabolic threshold is met.

BFR training causes greater recruitment of fast-twitch muscle fibers with light weight (i.e., 30% of a 1RM) similar to lifting heavy weight. This has caused some scientists to suggest it's the recruitment of fast-twitch fibers amplifying muscle growth.[65] A 2021 meta-analysis of BFR training found that it's an effective form of resistance exercise training for those injured with minimal risk and unable to perform traditional resistance exercise. BFR in medical studies was found to have no adverse impact in patients with heart and renal disease.[66] BFR training is great for stimulating muscle growth in patients with limited physical exertion. Another interesting fact, BFR training does not have to be taken to failure; a study comparing BFR training to failure with BFR training stopping short of failure resulted in similar muscle growth, despite the BFR group training until failure experiencing more pain.[67] Heavy weight training, which also causes greater recruitment of type II fibers, does not need to be taken to failure and can also result in muscle growth similar to training to failure. Another interesting finding is that BFR training to failure results in more damage than non-failure BFR training. This should remind you that *excessive muscle damage* is not the objective of your workout. When BFR train-

---

64 Charlie J. Davids et al., "Similar Morphological and Functional Training Adaptations Occur Between Continuous and Intermittent Blood Flow Restriction," *Journal of Strength and Conditioning Research* 35, no. 7 (July 1, 2021): 1784–93.

65 J. P. Loenneke et al., "Blood Flow Restriction: The Metabolite/Volume Threshold Theory," *Medical Hypotheses* 77, no. 5 (November 2011): 748–52.

66 Bradley C. Miller et al., "The Systemic Effects of Blood Flow Restriction Training: A Systematic Review," *International Journal of Sports Physical Therapy* 16, no. 4 (August 2, 2021): 978–90.

67 Manoel E. Lixandrão et al., ~Magnitude of Muscle Strength and Mass Adaptations Between High-Load Resistance Training Versus Low-Load Resistance Training Associated with Blood-Flow Restriction: A Systematic Review and Meta-Analysis," *Sports Medicine (Auckland, N.Z.)* 48, no. 2 (February 2018): 361–78.

ing is taken to failure, there is a delayed muscle growth response compared to non-failure training, indicative of excess muscle damage. Interestingly, there was no increase in muscle growth early in the study, with excessive muscle damage suggesting suppressed muscle growth compared to BFR training not to failure.[68] BFR is great to experiment with because it gives the joints, tendons, and ligaments a break from heavy lifting while providing a potent muscle growth stimulus. Before experimenting with BFR training, one should consult a qualified coach or professional to perform BFR training properly.

CHAPTER SUMMARY:

- Blood flow restriction (BFR) training and moderately heavy weight programs (>65% of a 1-RM) result in similar increases in muscle growth.

- When taken to failure, continuous tension (no lockouts) with lighter weight can build muscle similarly to a heavier weight with a lockout.

- Blood Flow Restriction training can be effective for increasing muscle growth.

- BFR training with taking off a cuff during rest resulted in similar increases in muscle growth as BFR being left on the entire time.

- BFR training to failure causes more muscle damage and inflammation than BFR stopping short of failure.

Increased muscle tension is required for adaptations to both strength and lean mass. Body weight exercises can result in tension on the muscle, but

---

68 Manoel E. Lixandrão et al., ~Magnitude of Muscle Strength and Mass Adaptations Between High-Load Resistance Training Versus Low-Load Resistance Training Associated with Blood-Flow Restriction: A Systematic Review and Meta-Analysis," *Sports Medicine (Auckland, N.Z.)* 48, no. 2 (February 2018): 361–78.

there is no change in the external resistance, as you can change with resistance exercise. Many body weight workouts have claimed to be superior to traditional resistance exercise for building strength and muscle mass.

MUSCLEGATE: BODY WEIGHT EXERCISES ARE THE BEST WAY TO INCREASE MUSCLE GROWTH

THE TRUTH EXPOSED: With the recent COVID-19 pandemic, more people are exercising at home. Compared to traditional resistance exercises, body weight exercises without progressive overload are inferior for increases in strength.[69] It's suggested that since body weight is the external resistance, repetitions are the only variable to change. It suggests that body weight exercises will eventually fail to provide the necessary tension to increase muscle growth. Beginners can increase muscle and strength with body weight exercises; however, advanced lifters will need a greater stimulus to increase tension. Here is an example of how you can provide a greater tension with different changes in body position while doing the push-up. Researchers analyzed the effects of different body weight push-up positions with changes in training load as a percentage of body mass. The results are:

- Push-up with your hands elevated on a 60cm block, 41% of your body weight

- Push-up on your knees, 49% of your body weight

- Push-up with your hands elevated on a 30 cm block, 55% of your body weight

- Full Push-up, 65% of your body weight,

---

69 Thomai Tsourlou et al., "The Effects of a Calisthenics and a Light Strength Training Program on Lower Limb Muscle Strength and Body Composition in Mature Women," *Journal of Strength and Conditioning Research* 17, no. 3 (August 2003): 590–98.

- Push-up with your feet elevated on 30 cm block, 70% of body weight

- Push-up with your feet elevated on a 60 cm block, 74% of your body weight.

This is an example of a push-up progression for beginners to gradually increase tension on the muscle based on your body weight.[70]

It's being found that if external resistance that increases tension overload is utilized with body weight exercises such as elastic bands during push-ups, similar increases in strength can be achieved as resistance exercise.[71] In this study, subjects either did bench press or push-ups with elastic bands that were progressively increased in tension for five weeks. The study found that both exercises increased muscle activation similarly to exercises as well as muscle strength. Muscle growth can occur if you progressively increase the tension with body weight exercises. For example, one study used a progressive push-up protocol in which the pushup was made harder each week. The subjects started with a wall pushup and gradually progressed to more difficult positions, such as a kneeling pushup, a full pushup, and a one-arm pushup. At the end of the study, the progressive push-up had similar strength and muscle size increases as those who performed the bench press.[72] It has also been shown that adding bands to your resistance exercise training can boost strength compared to resistance training alone.[73] TRX or suspension training is also a great alternative for

---

70 William P. Ebben et al., "Kinetic Analysis of Several Variations of Push-Ups," *The Journal of Strength & Conditioning Research* 25, no. 10 (October 2011): 2891–94.

71 Joaquin Calatayud et al., "Bench Press and Push-up at Comparable Levels of Muscle Activity Results in Similar Strength Gains," *Journal of Strength and Conditioning Research* 29, no. 1 (January 2015): 246–53..

72 Christopher Kotarsky et al., "Effect of Progressive Calisthenic Push-Up Training On Muscle Strength and Thickness," *Journal of Strength and Conditioning Research* 32 (March 1, 2018): 1.

73 Corey E. Anderson, Gary A. Sforzo, and John A. Sigg, "The Effects of Combining Elastic and Free Weight Resistance on Strength and Power in Athletes," *Journal of Strength and Conditioning Research* 22, no. 2 (March 2008): 567–74.

home workouts, as it has been found to increase muscle growth similar to resistance training.[74] In sum, body weight exercises have generally been found to lack the capacity to increase tension every week; however, a progressive loading bodyweight program that incorporates more tension can increase muscle mass.

THERE ARE MANY DIFFERENT WAYS TO INCREASE TENSION

When most people think of increasing tension, they think about adding more weight. There are several ways to increase tension by changing many training variables. Changing load (i.e., weight), proximity to failure, frequency, exercise selection, range of motion, technical execution of the exercise, and rest periods can all influence the potency of the exercise stimulus achieved with any given number of sets. Exercise intensity or % of a person's 1 Repetition Maximum (maximum weight a person can lift once) and volume (sets and repetitions) share an inverse relationship. Increasing one variable will come at the cost of the other. When the volume (sets and reps) goes up, intensity (weight) must go down and vice versa. Exercise difficulty increases as resistance exercise intensity (expressed as a percentage of 1RM) increases with high-intensity exercise compared to moderate and low-intensity exercise when similar rest periods are taken, despite decreasing repetitions and total workload.[75] If you want to add sets, you won't be able to train at higher intensities because of fatigue. If you examine the workout of the former six-time Mr. Olympia Dorian Yates, he trained with extremely high-intensity exercise but did very few sets. Fatigue increases as training intensities go up, and longer recovery is required with higher

---

74 Samuel Domingos Soligon et al., "Suspension Training vs. Traditional Resistance Training: Effects on Muscle Mass, Strength and Functional Performance in Older Adults," *European Journal of Applied Physiology* 120, no. 10 (October 2020): 2223–32.

75 Meghan L. Day et al., "Monitoring Exercise Intensity during Resistance Training Using the Session RPE Scale," *Journal of Strength and Conditioning Research* 18, no. 2 (May 2004): 353–58.

intensity exercise. It is impossible to gain muscle without some fatigue, but the key is to *manage fatigue* over the weeks during a training cycle. When excess fatigue accumulates over a period in your workouts, it is a good sign to back off. Adding reps, sets, and volume too fast can cause sub-optimal muscle growth because of accumulated stress and fatigue too quickly. As you will learn in Chapter 4, muscle growth is more than just adding weight to the bar; it's more about providing progressive overload followed by a period of recovery.

MEASURING EXERCISE INTENSITY

Over the past decade, an enormous amount of research has been conducted on tension overload and muscle growth. Throughout this book, you will notice that many studies use what is called a % Repetition Maximum (RM). A 1RM is the maximum weight you can lift for one repetition. For example, 60% of a 1RM would mean using 60% of the heaviest weight you could lift.

*Many studies use a % 1RM to examine muscle growth in response to different training intensities. You should regularly gauge your client's strength if you are a personal trainer. Performing a 1RM is not without risk; it's daunting to have a person lift as much weight as possible one time; therefore, there are alternative equations to estimate a person's 1RM. There are many equations to predict a person's maximal strength. The most popular prediction equation is the Brzycki formula for testing a person's 1RM. It's been validated to be fairly accurate as an alternative to a 1RM.[76]

---

76 Matheus Amarante do Nascimento et al., "Validation of the Brzycki Equation for the Estimation of 1RM in the Bench Press," *Revista Brasileira de Medicina Do Esporte* 13 (January 1, 2007): 40e–42e.

Brzycki formula for testing a person's 1RM: **weight / (1.0278 – 0.0278 × reps)**

Example of a bench press 10 RM: 225/ (1.0278-0.0278 X 10)

1RM Bench Press=300 lbs.

It should be mentioned that when testing with this prediction equation, the further you are from a true 1RM, the less reliable the formula becomes. It's recommended that you keep the repetitions less than 10 for predicting a person's 1RM for reliability.[77]

For the past decade, it's been advocated that lifting with heavier weight causes a greater increase in protein synthesis, leading to larger gains in muscle mass. Recent research suggests that protein synthesis increases with exercise intensity, but only up to a certain point, and then no further increases occur.

MUSCLEGATE: MAXIMAL WEIGHTS INCREASE MUSCLE PROTEIN SYNTHESIS.

THE TRUTH EXPOSED: In response to resistance exercise, provided all essential amino acids are consumed after exercise, protein synthesis increases, whereas protein breakdown remains the same. This process of repeated tension overload with increases in muscle protein synthesis 'drives' adaptations to exercise training. It was once thought that exercise intensities above 60% were necessary for optimal increases in muscle protein synthesis. Keep in mind that there is no direct correlation between the amount of weight (i.e., ~30-90% of a 1RM) you use and muscle growth

---

77 Jeff M. Reynolds, Toryanno J. Gordon, and Robert A. Robergs, "Prediction of One Repetition Maximum Strength from Multiple Repetition Maximum Testing and Anthropometry," *Journal of Strength and Conditioning Research* 20, no. 3 (August 2006): 584–92.

when sets are taken to complete failure.[78] Light-weight, high-volume resistance exercise (24 reps at 30% of a 1 RM to failure) is more effective at increasing muscle protein synthesis than heavy-weight, low-volume resistance exercise (5 reps at 90% of a 1 RM to failure). Interestingly, the 30% of a 1 RM-to-failure protocol induced similar increases in muscle protein synthesis to the 90% of a 1 RM to failure protocol at 4 hours post-exercise, but this response was sustained at 24 hours only in the 30% of a 1RM to failure group.[79] This study should not be misinterpreted to train with light weight all the time. *These studies suggest you can train with a lighter weight and get similar increases in muscle protein synthesis from a large range of exercise intensities, provided they are performed to failure.* Contrary to this, heavier weights can cause large increases in protein synthesis without being taken to failure. Researchers had subjects exercise at different exercise intensities that ranged from 20% to 90% of a 1RM. The study was designed to make the total exercise volume as close as possible between exercise intensities. Exercise intensity, sets, and reps for the groups were: 20% of 1-RM (3 sets × 27 reps), 40% (3 sets × 14 reps), 60% (3 sets × 9 reps), 75% (3 sets × 8 reps), and 90% (6 sets × 3 reps). Keep in mind; this study did not have subjects train to complete failure. *At the end of the study, protein synthesis maxed out at approximately 60% of a 1RM; adding higher amounts of weight did not result in additional increases in protein synthesis.* There was no difference in protein synthesis rates between 60%-90% of a 1RM.[80] **Despite the subjects not training to failure, heavier weights (>60% of a 1RM) can still maximally increase protein synthesis rates.** These studies suggest that with lighter weight (i.e., ~30% of a 1RM) sets should be taken to complete

---

78 Brad J. Schoenfeld et al., "Strength and Hypertrophy Adaptations Between Low – vs. High-Load Resistance Training: A Systematic Review and Meta-Analysis," *Journal of Strength and Conditioning Research* 31, no. 12 (December 2017): 3508–23.

79 Nicholas A. Burd et al., "Low-Load High Volume Resistance Exercise Stimulates Muscle Protein Synthesis More than High-Load Low Volume Resistance Exercise in Young Men," *PloS One* 5, no. 8 (August 9, 2010): e12033.

80 Vinod Kumar et al., "Age-Related Differences in the Dose-Response Relationship of Muscle Protein Synthesis to Resistance Exercise in Young and Old Men," *The Journal of Physiology* 587, no. 1 (January 15, 2009): 211–17.

muscular failure to maximize protein synthesis; however, heavier weights (i.e., 60-90% of a 1RM) do not need to be taken to complete failure and can still achieve maximal increases in protein synthesis.

Protein synthesis and its relation to muscle growth are complex bio-chemical processes that take place over time. Be cautious when extrap-olating acute protein synthesis studies to increases in muscle growth. It would seem logical to assume acute increases in protein synthesis correlate with muscle growth; however, there is evidence that acute protein synthe-sis levels are not correlated with muscle growth. A study by Mitchell et al. had men follow a linear periodized resistance training program consisting of 3 sets of 12 repetitions to 4 sets of 6 repetitions for 16 weeks. At the end of the study, despite increased muscle protein synthesis post-exercise and 6-hour post-exercise, the increases in muscle protein synthesis were not predictive of muscle hypertrophy.[81] It's likely that the protein synthe-sis responses are highly variable among lifters, and long-term changes in muscle protein synthesis may change over a training program. Keep this study in mind when you read a study that finds a particular exercise or sup-plement results in acute increases in protein synthesis; this does not mean it will translate into greater muscle growth. In sum, you can get optimal increases in protein synthesis from an extensive range of exercise inten-sities (i.e., 30-90%) provided the repetitions are close to failure; however, going heavier than 60% of a 1-RM will not elevate protein synthesis further based on the research.

---

81 Cameron J. Mitchell et al., "Acute Post-Exercise Myofibrillar Protein Synthesis Is Not Correlated with Resistance Training-Induced Muscle Hypertrophy in Young Men," *PLOS ONE* 9, no. 2 (February 24, 2014): e89431.

WEIGHT, MUSCULAR FAILURE, AND MUSCLE GROWTH

Scientists once believed that a weight had to be greater than 60% of a 1RM to stimulate muscle growth; this was known as the *hypertrophy zone*. It was stated in just about every journal that muscle growth occurs between 60-80% of a 1RM, with 8-12 repetitions. However, now we know that this is no longer true. Muscle growth can occur with both heavy (90% of a 1RM) and light weight (30% of a 1RM), provided the light weight reps are taken close to proximity to failure, and the volume is sufficient. In a meta-analysis of 23 studies with over 563 participants, it was found that muscle hypertrophy takes place with a wide spectrum of weights (i.e., 30 to 90% 1RM), and muscle failure seems to be an important component. The author also stated that heavy weight training to failure is demanding on the joints and tendons, possibly increasing the risks of overtraining. Thus, alternating periods with light, moderate, and heavy weight, is best for increasing muscle mass while minimizing excessive strain on the joints.[82]

So why does the weight not matter for muscle growth when the repetitions are taken to complete muscular failure? This is because of what is called Henneman's size principle.[83] This principle states that muscle fibers are recruited from the smallest to the largest. Small, slow-twitch are used first, but as the repetitions get more difficult, the muscle recruits more fast-twitch fibers. When using a light weight, as the slow-twitch muscle becomes fatigued, more and more fast-twitch muscle fibers are recruited. When training to failure with a light weight, all muscle fibers are fully activated at the end of a set. Using a lighter weight takes longer for the fast-twitch fibers to be recruited. It was once thought that the recruitment of

---

82 Marcio Lacio et al., "Effects of Resistance Training Performed with Different Loads in Untrained and Trained Male Adult Individuals on Maximal Strength and Muscle Hypertrophy: A Systematic Review," *International Journal of Environmental Research and Public Health* 18, no. 21 (January 2021): 11237.

83 E. Henneman, "Relation between Size of Neurons and Their Susceptibility to Discharge," *Science (New York, N.Y.)* 126, no. 3287 (December 27, 1957): 1345–47.

fast-twitch muscle fibers with weights above 60% of a 1RM was the key to muscle growth, but this is debatable. It has been found that training with a light weight (i.e., 30% of a 1RM) to failure can cause full muscle fiber recruitment; however, heavy weight (i.e., 70% of a 1RM) caused a larger recruitment of muscle fibers.[84] Training with heavy weight, light weight training at fast speeds, and light weight until failure all recruit fast-twitch fibers, but only training with heavy weights and light weights taken to failure results in muscle growth. For example, plyometrics incorporate fast explosive movement (i.e., drop jumps and bouncing exercises), recruit fast-twitch muscle fibers, and incorporate few reps resulting in sup-optimal muscle growth.[85] This possibly can be due to insufficient tension placed on the muscle for adequate periods. It could be that the plyometric training programs did not have enough volume to stimulate muscle growth. Researchers found that 8 weeks of plyometric training (explosive training such as box jumps, bounding exercises, jump squats) consisting of 24 sessions performed three times per week, with a total of 5,228 jumps, resulted in substantial muscle growth. Single fiber muscle cross sectional area increased in type I fibers by 23%, type IIa by 22+, and +30% in type IIa/IIx fibers.[86]

There must be a certain amount of fatigue for muscle growth to occur. Scientists now realize that it is less about how much weight is on the bar but more effort level. In a paper published titled, "Training for strength and hypertrophy: an evidence-based approach," which was published in *Current Opinion in Physiology*, the researchers placed the order of importance for muscle growth as Intensity of Effort > Volume > Training

84 Tyler W. D. Muddle et al., "Effects of Fatiguing, Submaximal High – versus Low-Torque Isometric Exercise on Motor Unit Recruitment and Firing Behavior," *Physiological Reports* 6, no. 8 (April 2018): e13675.

85 Jozo Grgic, Brad J. Schoenfeld, and Pavle Mikulic, "Effects of Plyometric vs. Resistance Training on Skeletal Muscle Hypertrophy: A Review," *Journal of Sport and Health Science*, June 21, 2020.

86 Laurent Malisoux et al., "Stretch-Shortening Cycle Exercises: An Effective Training Paradigm to Enhance Power Output of Human Single Muscle Fibers," *Journal of Applied Physiology (Bethesda, Md.: 1985)* 100, no. 3 (March 2006): 771–79.

Frequency > Daily Protein Intake > Inter-Set Rest Periods. If you notice, weight or load is not listed among the top principles for stimulating muscle growth, and it's the *intensity of effort*. This assumes that when light weight sets (30% of a 1RM) are taken to failure, it results in similar muscle growth as heavier weight (80%). The authors stated that if sets are performed at a high exertion level and taken too close to failure, weight is not as important as the effort.[87]

It should be mentioned that not all PhDs believe in the philosophy of just using effort level to build muscle. Some believe you still need to train with heavier weights. An editorial to the previous review by Dr. Juneau stated:

1. Load or weight does mediate resistance trained-induced muscular hypertrophy.

2. Progression in load should remain a variable of major focus for athletes looking to increase hypertrophy over a long period.

3. Lifting in the 'higher-load' (>70% 1RM) range should be emphasized in hypertrophy recommendations for healthy athletes, as it is more efficient.[88]

This again points to a combination of heavy and light weights for optimal increases in muscle growth. In the book *The Muscle & Strength Pyramids*,[89] written by Dr. Eric Helms, he recommends:

66%-75% of sets in the 6–12 rep range

25-33% of sets in the 1-6 rep range and 12-20 rep range.

---

87 Robert W Morton, Lauren Colenso-Semple, and Stuart M Phillips, "Training for Strength and Hypertrophy: An Evidence-Based Approach," *Current Opinion in Physiology*, Exercise Physiology, 10 (August 1, 2019): 90–95.

88 Carl-Etienne Juneau and Lucas Tafur, "Over Time, Load Mediates Muscular Hypertrophy in Resistance Training," *Current Opinion in Physiology*, Physiology of Pain, 11 (October 1, 2019): 147–48.

89 Helms, E., Valdez, A., Morgan, A. The Muscle and Strength Pyramids: Training, 2015.

CHAPTER SUMMARY:

- Muscle fibers can increase in size (diameter) or increase in length.

- High muscular tension, sufficient time exposure to that tension,

- and sufficient effort is required for muscle growth.

- Repetitions should be completed through a full range of motion.

- Type I fibers have the least potential for muscle growth. Type II has a greater capacity for muscle growth.

- Training at 30, 40%, 60%, or 80% of one-repetition maximum 1RM led to similar muscle growth when training to muscular failure.

- There is no direct correlation between the amount of weight you use and muscle growth when sets are taken to complete failure.

- Acute protein synthesis rates do not always correlate with long term muscle growth

CHAPTER 3

INTENSITY OF EFFORT DURING EACH SET

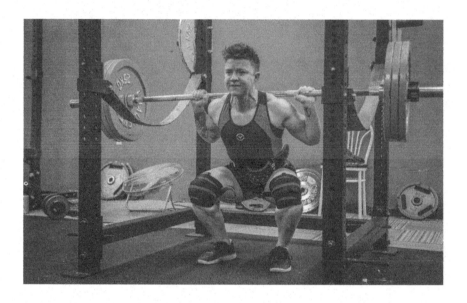

Mike Mentzer was a bodybuilder in the '80s who recommended *High-Intensity Training*. In my opinion, he was ahead of his time and understood that repetitions must be taken to the point of absolute failure to stimulate muscle growth. Some concepts, such as training one to two sets per bodypart, were misguided, but he understood the relationship between exercise intensity and recovery. Mentzer advocated low reps (6-9 reps), heavy weights, training to complete muscular failure, and adequate recovery (i.e., brief, infrequent workouts). He also advocated one to two sets per bodypart because he understood that high-intensity training resulted in fatigue, and therefore very few sets could be performed without overtraining. This was before there was any research on intensity and muscle growth. Still, he understood that exercise must reach a certain intensity or effort threshold to stimulate muscle growth and sets that stopped short of an intensity threshold were not as effective for muscle growth. He also understood that taking muscle groups to failure resulted in increased muscle damage and fatigue, so workouts were limited to one bodypart per week. He realized that training a muscle before it was fully recovered resulted in impaired workout performance the following workout. Although, it's known that all sets do not need to be taken to failure for muscle growth (Chapter 7). Both light weight taken to failure and heavy weight stopping a few reps short of failure stimulates muscle growth equally. Mentzer was correct that exercise intensity must reach a certain threshold for muscle growth to occur.

NOT ALL REPS PRODUCE MUSCLE GROWTH

Keep in mind that you can keep adding sets to your workout and still not gain muscle. You must train close to the point of muscular failure to generate muscle growth. If you stop when your muscle starts fatiguing, you are not maximizing muscle growth. The first few reps do not stimulate muscle growth, whereas the final few reps with effort are called *stimulating reps*. Therefore, not all reps produce muscle growth; only those with sufficient exercise effort are the muscle growing reps. *It's been suggested that the last 5 reps at the end of a set are the most effective for muscle growth.* The last 5 reps from failure are where full motor unit or full muscle fiber activation occurs. A 5 RM translates to about 85% of a 1RM, which is enough weight to force maximum muscle fiber activation with every repetition. During the last 3-5 reps before failure, a plateau in muscle fiber activation occurs, meaning the muscle fiber has been fully activated.[90] For example, light weight (i.e., 20% of a 1RM) resistance exercise stopping short of failure

---

90 Emil Sundstrup et al., "Muscle Activation Strategies during Strength Training with Heavy Loading vs. Repetitions to Failure," *Journal of Strength and Conditioning Research* 26, no. 7 (July 2012): 1897–1903.

fails to produce muscle growth. This is due to a low amount of stimulating reps being performed. The stimulating reps will only occur during the last few reps in conjunction with a high level of effort and fatigue. Conversely, doing maximal strength tests every day fails to produce muscle growth because of a low number of stimulating reps.

As the research has shown, you can still grow muscle by using heavier weights; you need more sets to increase the number of stimulating reps. This was demonstrated in the Schoenfeld study mentioned earlier in which both heavy and light weights equally increased muscle growth when the volume is similar. It is much easier to achieve more stimulating reps with a moderate to heavy weight than a light weight taken close to failure. This can explain why *SuperSlow, although capable of stimulating muscle growth, are less effective than moderate weights/heavier weights because SuperSlow involves a low amount of* stimulating reps. This means most of the reps you are doing are not stimulating muscle growth because the tension is low, and very few type II fibers are being recruited. In comparison, training with a heavier weight to failure results in more stimulating reps faster. You can train with either ten reps to failure or 20 reps to failure and get equal muscle growth because both incorporate stimulating reps as long as the volume is sufficient. Subjects training with 24–28 repetitions with a light weight (30% 1-RM) gained a similar amount of muscle to those training with 8–12 repetitions with a moderate weight (70% 1-RM) when all sets are taken to complete muscular failure and volume is similar.[91] *It's important to reiterate that it's been estimated that the final five reps performed to failure are the most important reps for stimulating muscle growth.*

---

91 Daniel Kapsis et al., "Changes in Body Composition and Strength after 12 Weeks of High-Intensity Functional Training with Two Different Loads in Physically Active Men and Women: A Randomized Controlled Study," *Sports* 10 (January 4, 2022): 7.

DON'T COUNT WARM-UP SETS

There is a term called *junk volume*. This means you are adding sets but not meeting the minimum expectations for exercise intensity. Repetitions performed with insufficient weight, which do not meet a high-intensity threshold, do not stimulate muscle growth. Warm-up sets and sets that are performed in excess that do not meet the required intensity for muscle growth are considered junk volume. Warm up sets are important; just don't count them as muscle building sets. It's not uncommon for some Instagram fitness models to brag about their 2-hour workout. How much of those sets meets the minimum threshold for intensity after the first hour? More than likely, most of the ultra-marathon workouts incorporate a large amount of junk volume. Any repetition that is not in the threshold of the 5-rep range away from failure is not conducive for muscle growth.

Warming up with light weights to get the muscles and joints ready for heavier weight should not be included as regular sets because there are *no stimulating reps*. Another example of junk volume would be that if you are training a body part once a week and doing 30 sets for chest total. By the time you get to those last few sets at the end of the workout, you will be significantly fatigued, and the intensity threshold may not be big enough to stimulate muscle growth. It would be much wiser to do ten sets broken up into three sessions over the week than try to do one workout. Therefore, training a body part once per week is not the best way to train because the fatigue is too great. Trying to perform an entire week's training in one day will lead to increased fatigue and excessive junk volume, which will inevitably lead to reduced gains in strength and lean mass. The sets performed in the latter part of the workout will not be as effective as if you were to cut the workout in half and perform it later in the week. Excessive sets performed in any one workout will lead to diminished exercise intensity, resulting in junk volume. An example of junk volume would be the study by Haun et al., in which subjects gradually increased their set volume until they performed 30 sets per bodypart. Still, the mean average of the group showed no further increases in muscle growth after 20 sets.[92] Another example of junk volume is the German Volume Training study in which 5 sets of 10 repetitions in the squats resulted in greater increases in lean mass in the legs than 10 sets of 10 repetitions.[93] These studies suggest that sets beyond a certain point led to no further increases in muscle growth. The optimal number of sets for muscle growth will be discussed in Chapter 5.

EXERCISE EFFORT MUST BE OF SUFFICIENT EFFORT FOR MUSCLES TO GROW

High threshold muscle fibers that are capable of muscle growth are only recruited when the sets are taken close to failure. It's commonly suggested that if you have five reps left in you and you stop short, you will not build much muscle because you are stopping when fast-twitch fibers, which are most capable of muscle growth, are just starting to be maximally recruited. To give you an example, researchers measured velocity loss during sets. As you get fatigued, your muscles can't move the weight as fast, and velocity or how fast you lift a weight decreases. Subjects stopped each set of squats after a 20% or a 40% velocity loss in the set. The group that trained with 40% velocity loss was training closer to failure. At the end of the study, the group that trained closer to failure had more muscle growth than the group that trained further away from failure (20% velocity loss).[94] The 40% group consistently felt they were training closer to failure most of the time, while the 20% group felt they could have performed additional reps. This points to that training must be closer to the proximity of muscular failure for muscle growth.

---

92 Cody T. Haun et al., "Effects of Graded Whey Supplementation During Extreme-Volume Resistance Training," *Frontiers in Nutrition* 5 (2018): 84.

93 Daniel A. Hackett et al., "Effects of a 12-Week Modified German Volume Training Program on Muscle Strength and Hypertrophy-A Pilot Study," *Sports (Basel, Switzerland)* 6, no. 1 (January 29, 2018): E7.

94 F. Pareja-Blanco et al., "Effects of Velocity Loss during Resistance Training on Athletic Performance, Strength Gains and Muscle Adaptations," *Scandinavian Journal of Medicine & Science in Sports* 27, no. 7 (July 2017): 724–35.

ARE YOU TRAINING AT FULL EXERCISE INTENSITY?

Many people think they exert full effort in the gym, but this may not truly be the case. One study asked 160 men who regularly exercised and asked them, "What was the weight you can normally bench press for 10 repetitions?" The subjects were allowed to warm up and then do their self-selected weight. On average, the subjects did 16 reps when they said they could only bench press the weight 10 times.[95] The lead author of the study stated, "*It was concluded that most individuals can perform a number of repetitions well above the 10 repetitions predicted for the selected load. Therefore, the training routines are not compatible with maximum effort or with their most prevalent goal, muscle hypertrophy.*" If you recall from the previous section, the last 5 reps before failure are the most important for muscle growth. These participants did 6 more reps than they normally performed. This suggests that most people are not training at their full exercise effort. Here is a study that will blow your mind! Researchers had subjects train biceps and used one arm with weights using a load of 70% 1RM. The other arm was trained with no weights but required participants to contract their bicep "as hard as possible" throughout the full range of motion of each repetition. After the 6-week training period, both arms increased in muscle size.[96] Muscle growth occurred without any external weight, only contracting the arm as hard as possible. It may be the case for higher effort during exercise instead of adding more weight. It seems wise to suggest that if you are looking to increase muscle growth, squeezing the muscle as hard as you can increase the intensity of effort with each repetition.

---

95 Sebastião Barbosa-Netto, Obanshe S. d~Acelino-e-Porto, and Marcos B. Almeida, ~Self-Selected Resistance Exercise Load: Implications for Research and Prescription," *The Journal of Strength & Conditioning Research* 35 (February 2021): S166.

96 Brittany R. Counts et al., "The Acute and Chronic Effects of 'NO LOAD' Resistance Training," *Physiology & Behavior* 164, no. Pt A (October 1, 2016): 345–52.

HIGH INTENSITY EXERCISE MAY BOOST ANDROGEN RECEPTORS

Since we are on the topic of intensity, although this is highly controversial, high-intensity exercise or heavy weight may boost androgen receptors. The androgen receptor is what circulating testosterone binds to and activates protein synthesis. Think of a store looking to get as many people as possible in the store for sales (i.e., muscle growth). The store will not have a very successful business if the parking lot is too small. If the store's parking lot has a max capacity of ten parking spots (few androgen receptors), fewer people (i.e., testosterone) will go into the store. Now think of the same parking lot with 50 parking spots (more androgen receptors). Many more cars can be parked in those spots, and more business will occur. The same concept applies to testosterone and androgen receptors on the muscle; more androgen receptors can result in more testosterone having a greater physiological response. Studies have found that people with more androgen receptors have greater muscle mass.[97] One study found that heavy weight resistance exercises increased androgen receptors post-exercise. In contrast, the light weight group had no effect.[98] Although we know that both heavy and light weight training can produce similar muscle growth, it points out that different intensities of training can have different molecular effects on the muscle. Your chest may grow well with a certain number of sets, and your calves may not, despite doing the same sets. It could be because of more androgen receptors in the chest, causing greater muscle growth. It's been found that there is a direct correlation between the increases in androgen receptors and muscle growth. In contrast, post-exercise changes in testosterone were

---

97 Robert W. Morton et al., "Muscle Androgen Receptor Content but Not Systemic Hormones Is Associated With Resistance Training-Induced Skeletal Muscle Hypertrophy in Healthy, Young Men," *Frontiers in Physiology* 9 (2018): 1373.

98 Thomas D. Cardaci et al., "High-Load Resistance Exercise Augments Androgen Receptor-DNA Binding and Wnt/β-Catenin Signaling without Increases in Serum/Muscle Androgens or Androgen Receptor Content," *Nutrients* 12, no. 12 (December 15, 2020): E3829.

not found to have an effect.[99] Others have found that overtraining reduces androgen receptor concentrations in muscle.[100] Tension overload on the muscle influences increasing androgen receptors.[101] This again suggests that a combination of heavy and light weight can optimize muscle growth.

REPETITIONS IN RESERVE (REPS LEFT IN THE TANK)

Some researchers believe some sets should be taken to complete muscular failure, whereas others believe you should stop just short of failure. Lifters use what is called *repetitions in reserve* (RIR), which is the number of reps away from failure or reps left in the gas tank. One of the best metrics to use whether you are close to failure is rep speed velocity. A relationship exists between repetition velocity and proximity to failure.[102] If you watch a person lift the weight, you will notice a noticeable decrease in how fast the weight is moving towards the end of the set. This is where RIR begins. If you are doing a set of bench presses for eight repetitions, but you could have done two more reps before complete muscular failure, then your RIR or reps left in the gas tank is 2.

The biggest issue with gauging RIR (i.e., exercise intensity effort level) is that RIR is highly variable among subjects. Untrained lifters tend to *underpredict* how hard they are exercising and are more accurately able

99 Cameron J. Mitchell et al., "Muscular and Systemic Correlates of Resistance Training-Induced Muscle Hypertrophy," *PloS One* 8, no. 10 (2013): e78636.

100 Justin X. Nicoll et al., "MAPK, Androgen, and Glucocorticoid Receptor Phosphorylation Following High-Frequency Resistance Exercise Non-Functional Overreaching," *European Journal of Applied Physiology* 119, no. 10 (October 2019): 2237–53.

101 M. M. Bamman et al., "Mechanical Load Increases Muscle IGF-I and Androgen Receptor MRNA Concentrations in Humans," *American Journal of Physiology. Endocrinology and Metabolism* 280, no. 3 (March 2001): E383-390.

102 Javier Riscart-López et al., ~Effects of Four Different Velocity-Based Training Programming Models on Strength Gains and Physical Performance,~ *Journal of Strength and Conditioning Research* 35, no. 3 (March 1, 2021): 596–603.

to gauge how close they are to failure when fewer reps are performed.[103] This means that untrained lifters are more likely to know how close they are to true failure when doing a max set of 8 reps compared to a set of 30 reps. However, well-trained lifters are much more accurate in determining how close to failure they are.[104] One drawback of super high rep training (>30 reps) is that it's much harder to gauge whether you are training to complete muscular failure. For example, anyone that has ever done high repetition squats knows how exhausting it is on the body. Did you stop the set due to cardiovascular fatigue, or are you training your muscle to complete failure? For example, you can jump rope before a set of squats; it's not your leg muscles that are being taken to the point of failure, your heart rate is elevated, and your cardiovascular system is taxed rather than your muscles. The same concept applies with high rep squatting (> 30 reps); cardiovascular fatigue is more likely to stop the set than maximal muscle fatigue.

RIR is a valuable way to gauge your training progress; for example, if you start a program, the first few weeks should be easy and stick to an RIR of 3-4. As your exercise intensity increases, you want to be in the two or less RIR range. Before taking a break, the last week of training is when you can redline it and train to complete muscular failure (0 RIR). The muscle growth range has been recommended to be between 0-5. The reason 5 is the least number of repetitions one should stop is based on a 2019 study in which subjects were divided into four groups are shown below. The subjects reported how hard they were exercising in each group. Muscle growth increases are marked by percentages for the groups were the following:

- Repetitions to failure with low load (30% of a 1RM); ~34.4 repetitions) = +7.8%

---

103 Sean K. Mansfield et al., "Estimating Repetitions in Reserve for Resistance Exercise: An Analysis of Factors Which Impact on Prediction Accuracy," *Journal of Strength and Conditioning Research*, August 31, 2020.

104 Michael C. Zourdos et al., "Novel Resistance Training-Specific Rating of Perceived Exertion Scale Measuring Repetitions in Reserve," *Journal of Strength and Conditioning Research* 30, no. 1 (January 2016): 267–75.

- Repetitions to failure with high load (80% of a 1RM); ~12.4 repetitions) = +8.1%

- Repetitions not to failure with low load (30% of a 1RM); ~19.6 repetitions) = +2.8%

- Repetitions not to failure with high load (80% of a 1RM); ~6.7 repetitions) = +7.7%

All the groups, except those that used light weight and stopped short of failure (i.e., not a statistical increase in muscle growth compared to the other groups), gained roughly similar increases in muscle mass. All the failure groups had exertion or intensity of effort levels at max or close to max. The heavy load group that stopped short of failure average exercise level was about a 5 RIR (~80% of a 1RM). If you notice, the group that trained with 80% until failure averaged 12 repetitions, yet the group that used 80% and performed 7 repetitions (i.e., stopped 5 reps short of failure) gained the same amount of muscle mass. This suggests that 5 RIR should be the minimum that you stop short of failure for increasing muscle growth.[105] It should be emphasized this is a single study, but it suggests that 5 RIR is the minimum for muscle growth. Many of your sets should be in the 2-3 RIR range.

It does not matter what weight you are using either; whether you are doing reps of 20 or reps of 12, the last five reps seem to be the most critical for muscle growth. You can do certain things to psychologically push you closer to hitting your RIR numbers, such as listening to your favorite music, having a spotter, and reducing mental fatigue (i.e., discussed in Chapter 8). Typically, your RIR will drop by 1 RIR with each successive set. As you progress through your training cycle, fatigue is inevitable. Fatigue cannot be eliminated, but it can be managed.

---

105 Thiago Lasevicius et al., "Muscle Failure Promotes Greater Muscle Hypertrophy in Low-Load but Not in High-Load Resistance Training." *Journal of Strength and Conditioning Research*, December 27, 2019.

SAMPLE RIR SCALE

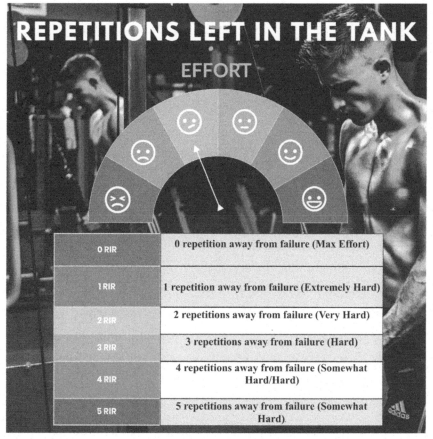

*Most of your repetitions for building muscle should be in the 2-3 RIR range.

TRAINED LIFTERS MAY BE ABLE TO TRAIN FURTHER AWAY FROM FAILURE

There is evidence that trained lifters can train with an intensity further away from failure and still make impressive gains in muscle growth. This is a highly controversial study, but researchers trained subjects with 80% of 1RM. The total volume was equal; one group trained with an estimated 5-7 RIR (far from failure), and the other group trained to complete muscular failure. At the end of the study, the group that trained further away from failure had the same muscle growth as a group training to failure.

Again, this is one study, but it suggests that advanced lifters may be able to train further away from failure; and still gain muscle! Other studies have replicated these findings by finding that training with a heavier weight and further away from failure (4+ RIR) can see similar growth to groups training closer to failure (0-3 RIR).[106] Keep in mind that training with a light weight (i.e., 30% of a 1RM) and avoiding failure results in inferior muscle growth. These studies provide valuable insights for those looking to manage workout fatigue; advanced lifters can train further away from failure while benefiting from increased recovery and muscle growth.

> *If you look at the research involving RIR, you could just ditch the training diary and keep RIR less than 3. As you know, muscle growth is more dependent on the level of effort and less on the weight on the bar and the reps. Muscle hypertrophy occurs with both light and heavy weight provided the intensity of effort is sufficiently high. If you are performing enough sets and using a full range of motion with suitable form, you may be able to train with 1-2 reps away from failure. Many repetitions can stimulate muscle growth if they are taken close to failure.
>
> *If you are a personal trainer, you should not only track their sets and reps but also monitor how hard they are exercising, such as I could have done 3-5 more reps (add more weight or reps next session), I could have done 1-2 more reps (i.e., sweet spot), that was extremely hard (i.e., back off the next set). The intensity of effort is an important variable for increasing muscle growth. When you start a new training cycle, start with around 4-5 reps in reserve, and as the volume increases, progress from 4-5 to approximately 0-1 the last week of your training.

---

106 Fernando Pareja-Blanco et al., "Effects of Velocity Loss in the Bench Press Exercise on Strength Gains, Neuromuscular Adaptations, and Muscle Hypertrophy," *Scandinavian Journal of Medicine & Science in Sports* 30, no. 11 (2020): 2154–66.

Starting a new training cycle with 0-1 RIR means the training stimulus is too high, leading to overtraining as the volume progresses. A recent study found that gradually increasing RIR over 12-weeks (i.e., 3 blocks) was superior to % of a 1RM for increasing strength despite using a similar training volume. In the RIR group, subjects in blocks one and two (weeks 1-8) increased RIR increased from 4 RIR in week one to 1 RIR in week four); in block three (weeks 9-12), they did sets that increased from 2 RIR in week nine to 0 RIR in week 12). The % 1RM group did sets with 65%-72.5% in block one; in block two, they used sets with 77.5%-85%; in block three, they did sets between 87.5%-95%. In each % 1RM block, there was a 2.5% increase per week. The difference between the groups was that the RIR group allowed the lifters to adjust loads based on how they were feeling on that day, whereas the %1RM had to train with a fixed weight that day. The group using RIR had superior increases in strength due to using heavier absolute loads over the 12-week training period. The RIR group increased front squats by 11.7% versus 8.3% with fixed loading. The RIR led to a 10.8% increase in strength compared to 7.1% for fixed loading for back squats.[107] Some of the superior strength increases using RIR were because of the ability to not use a maximal effort each set and not training to failure except in the last week of the training program. Remember that multi-joint exercises like the squat are more fatiguing than single-joint exercises like the machine preacher curl. It's more likely that you can train single-joint exercises like arm curls and triceps extensions to failure with less overall strain on the nervous system than taking multi-joint exercises like the squat and deadlift to muscular failure.

---

107 Timothy Graham and Daniel J. Cleather, "Autoregulation by 'Repetitions in Reserve' Leads to Greater Improvements in Strength Over a 12-Week Training Program Than Fixed Loading," *Journal of Strength and Conditioning Research* 35, no. 9 (September 1, 2021): 2451–56.

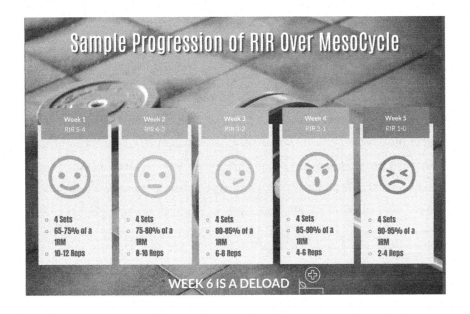

YOU CAN BUILD MUSCLE WITH A
WIDE RANGE OF REPETITIONS

It's recommended that for optimal muscle growth, you must use a wide variety of repetition ranges (6-30 repetitions). It's recommended that you keep reps greater than 6 for building muscle. For example, in a 2016 study, subjects trained with low reps, heavy weight (2-4 reps), or a bodybuilding program (8-12 reps) for eight weeks. Both groups completed each set to complete muscular failure. The heavy weight, low reps group had better strength gains, *but the bodybuilding group had double the muscle growth.*[108] In a 2019 study, subjects who trained to failure and were assigned to a high rep (20-25 repetition maximum) gained similar increases in muscle to those using low reps (6-8 repetition maximum); however, the heavy

---

108 Brad J. Schoenfeld et al., "Differential Effects of Heavy Versus Moderate Loads on Measures of Strength and Hypertrophy in Resistance-Trained Men," *Journal of Sports Science & Medicine* 15, no. 4 (December 1, 2016): 715–22.

weight groups had a slightly greater increase in muscle mass.[109] Another interesting finding was that the time under tension was 60-75 seconds for the high rep group. In contrast, the strength group TUT was 18-24 seconds. Despite the differences in TUT for both the groups, muscle growth was similar. Keep in mind that there is immediate recruitment of the fast-twitch muscle fibers when using heavier weights, whereas light weights will utilize most type I fibers. Still, as the muscle gets fatigued, more type II fibers will be recruited. By using a wide variety of repetition ranges, you get optimal recruitment of type I and type II fibers. As mentioned several times, you can build weight with light weight, but using high repetitions is psychologically tougher and generates more fatigue than moderate to heavy weight training.

MUSCLE ACTIVATION MAXES OUT
AT A CERTAIN THRESHOLD

It's well known that muscle activation increases with increasing exercise intensity. Therefore, light weight exercise taken to failure can stimulate muscle growth. This is due to the muscle fiber fatiguing, resulting in greater activation of Type II fibers similar to training with a heavy weight. Also, the same principles apply to BFR training, which uses a very light weight, but can increase muscle growth similar to heavy weight because of the high levels of fatigue and metabolic stress. Keep in mind that as you add more weight, muscle activation will not further increase at a certain point, and other muscle groups increase in activity. Your goal is to build muscle, not see how much you can lift in the gym.

A moderate weight can often result in more muscle activation and better exercise form. For example, researchers had subjects train on the bench press with 70%, 80%, 90%, and 100% of their 1RM. The Pec EMG

---

109 Salvador Vargas et al., "Comparison of Changes in Lean Body Mass with a Strength – versus Muscle Endurance-Based Resistance Training Program," *European Journal of Applied Physiology* 119, no. 4 (April 2019): 933–40.

(i.e., chest muscle activation) was maxed at about 70%, whereas over 70%, the anterior deltoid and triceps began taking over at higher weights. Interestingly, you have greater pec activity at 70% than 100%.[110] Similar findings have been found with the squat comparing 80%, 90%, and 100% of a 1RM. It was found that increases in muscle activation were seen only for vastus medialis and gluteus maximus during 90% and 100% of a 1RM, respectively, compared to those during 80%. There was no statistically significant difference in muscle activation between 90% and 100% for any muscle. Subjects using 100% RM resulted in a forward lean, which resulted in changes in hip joint kinematics. The author concluded that using 90% of a 1RM was safer and resulted in the same muscle activation as a 100% RM.[111] Caution should be emphasized by extrapolating "muscle activation" studies to muscle growth. There are no longitudinal studies to suggest increased "muscle activation" or increased EMG is predictive of muscle growth.[112] Jenkins et al. (2015) conducted an EMG study and found that, when taken to momentary muscular failure, 3 sets of 80% 1 RM caused greater muscle activation (i.e., greater EMG amplitude) than did 3 sets of 30% 1 RM. However, muscle growth increased in both groups.[113] This suggests that muscle activation is a poor method of predicting long-term muscle growth.

With experienced athletes, focusing on the muscle and actively "squeezing the muscle" can increase muscle activation of the arms and chest. Mentally focusing on a muscle has been found to increase the muscle

---

110 Henryk Król and Artur Gołaś, "Effect of Barbell Weight on the Structure of the Flat Bench Press," *Journal of Strength and Conditioning Research* 31, no. 5 (May 2017): 1321–37.

111 Hasan U. Yavuz and Deniz Erdag, "Kinematic and Electromyographic Activity Changes during Back Squat with Submaximal and Maximal Loading," *Applied Bionics and Biomechanics* 2017 (2017): 9084725.

112 Andrew D. Vigotsky et al., "Interpreting Signal Amplitudes in Surface Electromyography Studies in Sport and Rehabilitation Sciences," *Frontiers in Physiology* 8 (January 4, 2018): 985.

113 Nathaniel D. M. Jenkins et al., "Muscle Activation during Three Sets to Failure at 80 vs. 30 % 1RM Resistance Exercise," *European Journal of Applied Physiology* 115, no. 11 (November 1, 2015): 2335–47.

activation of these regions during the bench press at relative loads between 20 and 60% of a 1RM. However, mentally focusing on a muscle resulted in no greater muscle activation above 80% of a 1RM. The researchers found that selectively focusing on a muscle has a threshold between 60%-80% of a 1RM.[114] With that being said, more weight will cause more fatigue; it is best to keep the weight between 30-85% of a 1RM to stimulate muscle growth. Another option is to incorporate a system like Push/Pull Workouts, where muscle groups are organized around movements in which muscle groups involved in pushing movements are structured in one workout—allowing pulling muscle fibers to rest and be trained on a separate day. If you train chest and biceps on Monday, then on Tuesday, your back workout could be impacted by your biceps still being fatigued from the previous day's workout, which can lead to a reduction in volume the following day. As you will learn in Chapter 10, exercises that use opposing muscle groups are advantageous for increasing performance and reducing fatigue.

SAMPLE PUSH/PULL ROUTINE

DAY 1: "Push" workout: Train all the upper body pushing muscles, i.e., the chest, shoulders, and triceps. Example: bench press, incline press, military press, dips

DAY 2: "Pull" workout: you train all the upper body pulling muscles, i.e., the back and biceps. Example: Deadlifts, Lat pulldown, biceps curls

Day 3: "Legs" workout: you train the entire lower body, i.e., the quads, hamstrings, calves, and abdominals. Example: Squats, leg press, leg curls.

---

114 Joaquin Calatayud et al., "Importance of Mind-Muscle Connection during Progressive Resistance Training," *European Journal of Applied Physiology* 116, no. 3 (March 2016): 527–33.

DOES HEAVIER WEIGHT INCREASE MUSCLE GROWTH OF SPECIFIC FIBER TYPES?

Fiber-type proportion can vary by individual and is influenced by genetics and the type of training specificity.[115] It's suggested that training with a combination of heavy and light weight, both fiber types (Type I and Type II) can increase in size instead of just lifting heavy, which can only increase Type II fibers. Resistance training with heavier weights (i.e., ≥60% of a 1RM) emphasizes a greater growth of Type II muscle fibers, while resistance training with lighter weights (i.e., <60% of 1RM) might primarily augment hypertrophy of type I muscle fibers. Most lifters may neglect to increase type I fibers since they have a lower capacity to increase muscle size, but if you increase the size of type I fibers, the net result will be a bigger muscle.

Muscle biopsies of strength athletes always have more type II fibers. When comparing strength athletes such as Olympic weightlifters and powerlifters to bodybuilders, it was found that strength athletes who trained with heavier weight (>90% of a 1RM) had greater increases in type II fibers. In contrast, bodybuilders had equal hypertrophy of both types I and II fibers.[116] If you are strictly looking to put on muscle for aesthetic purposes, increasing the size of both Type I and Type II fibers will cause a greater total muscle mass. The question is," Should you try with light weight training to increase type I fibers?"

The evidence that training with light weights stimulates more growth of type I fibers is controversial. One study compared men who trained one leg with a heavy load (10 sets of eight repetitions at 70% of a 1 RM) and the other leg with a light load (10 sets of 36 repetitions at 15.5% of a 1 RM). There were no increases in muscle hypertrophy in type I fibers with

---

115 J. A. Simoneau and C. Bouchard, "Genetic Determinism of Fiber Type Proportion in Human Skeletal Muscle," *FASEB Journal: Official Publication of the Federation of American Societies for Experimental Biology* 9, no. 11 (August 1995): 1091–95.

116 Andrew C. Fry, "The Role of Resistance Exercise Intensity on Muscle Fibre Adaptations," *Sports Medicine (Auckland, N.Z.)* 34, no. 10 (2004): 663–79.

the light load training. Still, there was an 18% increase in satellite cells, revealing a new aspect of myogenic precursor cell activation.[117] It has been suggested that metabolic stress from light weight training can increase type I fiber growth.

CAN METABOLIC STRESS INCREASE TYPE I FIBER GROWTH?

The theory of training with light weight training to increase metabolic stress to increase muscle Type I fiber growth is highly controversial. For example, researchers had subjects train with heavy (6-10 reps) and light weight (20-30 reps) calf raises. If you train with light weights to increase type I fibers holds true, then the light weight group should have seen increases in Type I fibers. However, the increases in muscle growth were similar for all the muscles (Type I and II) independent of the weight used.[118] Based on most studies looking at changes in fiber types with light and heavy weight resistance training, there does not appear to be changes in muscle fiber types corresponding to high and low repetition training regimens.[119]

Still, some interesting studies suggest that metabolic stress may increase type I fiber growth. Powerlifters were randomized to a power-lifting protocol (60-85% of a 1RM) or a light weight powerlifting protocol (31% of a 1RM), combined with blood flow restriction training (i.e., a training method which impedes blood flow and results in high metabolic stress). The group performing low-load blood flow restriction training experienced significant quad hypertrophy, including preferential type

---

117 A. L. Mackey et al., "Myogenic Response of Human Skeletal Muscle to 12 Weeks of Resistance Training at Light Loading Intensity," *Scandinavian Journal of Medicine & Science in Sports* 21, no. 6 (December 2011): 773–82.

118 Brad J. Schoenfeld et al., "Do the Anatomical and Physiological Properties of a Muscle Determine Its Adaptive Response to Different Loading Protocols?," *Physiological Reports* 8, no. 9 (May 2020): e14427.

119 Jozo Grgic, "The Effects of Low-Load Vs. High-Load Resistance Training on Muscle Fiber Hypertrophy: A Meta-Analysis," *Journal of Human Kinetics* 74 (August 2020): 51–58.

I fiber growth (12%), while the group doing traditional, heavier training failed to grow.[120] Again, this is one study, but it could suggest that metabolic stress with light weight *may* increase type I fiber growth, but the evidence is very limited. Dr. Grgic, one of the leading experts in muscle hypertrophy, suggests that since aerobic exercise can result in increases in Type I fibers, he hypothesizes that a *greater time under load* with exercises taken to muscular failure might contribute to increases in Type I fiber.[121]

SAMPLE COMBINED TENSION, METABOLIC STRESS, MUSCLE DAMAGE WORKOUT

Reps		Rest Period
Tension	4 sets x 5 Reps	3-5 minutes
Metabolic Stress	4 sets x 20 Reps	<1 minute
(Super Sets, Drop Sets, Pre-Exhaustion Training, Rest-Pause)		
Muscle Damage	4 sets x 10 Reps	2-3 minutes
(Eccentric Exercise: Lifting with 2 legs, lowering with 1 leg)		

MUSCLEGATE: TO GROW YOUR CALVES, YOU NEED TO PERFORM > 20 REPS.

THE TRUTH EXPOSED: This is another gym fitness myth that has been around for decades. I am not sure how this myth was started, but I know that it's still around today. The "bro-science" or an unscientific rationale spoken by bodybuilders is that because the calves consist predominantly of slow-twitch muscle fibers, for them to grow, they need to be trained with high reps. This myth was debunked by muscle guru Dr. Brad Schoenfeld

---

120 Thomas Bjørnsen et al., ~Type 1 Muscle Fiber Hypertrophy after Blood Flow-Restricted Training in Powerlifters," *Medicine and Science in Sports and Exercise* 51, no. 2 (February 2019): 288–98.

121 Grgic, J., Homolak, J., Mikulic, P., Botella, J., & Schoenfeld, B. J. (2018). Inducing hypertrophic effects of type I skeletal muscle fibers: A hypothetical role of time under load in resistance training aimed at muscular hypertrophy. Medical hypotheses, 112, 40–42.

in 2020. Dr. Schoenfeld had subjects train their calves with a light weight (20–30 repetitions) and heavy weight (6–10 repetitions). The calf muscle has different regions that have different fiber type distributions. The medial and lateral gastrocnemius have an even combination of both slow-twitch and fast-twitch muscle fibers, while the soleus is mostly slow-twitch. So, if the soleus consists of type I fibers, it should have responded better to high rep training. The cool part about this study is that each subject trained one leg with high reps and the other leg with low reps. Each group was trained to complete muscular failure, and no bouncing was allowed during the repetitions. *At the end of the study, both the high-rep and low-rep training groups gained similar increases in muscle mass in the calf muscle.*[122] All three muscles responded similarly to the use of heavy and light weights. This suggests that both heavy and light weight can equally stimulate calf growth. One of the biggest mistakes that people commonly make is loading up the calf machine with weight and not using a full range of motion. The lifter will start bouncing up and down on the calf raise machine, doing partial reps. As you will read in Chapter 10, a full range of motion is needed to optimize muscle growth. Here is a calf training tip that may increase calf growth. Between sets, stretch the calf muscles between sets with just the weight with no movement. When subjects performed weight assisted calf stretches for 3 minutes, five days a week for six weeks, it resulted in a 5.6% increase in calf muscle growth.[123] This is controversial, but possibly more stretching can increase calf muscle growth. Another study found that when volleyball players stretched their calf muscles (i.e., static calf muscle stretch) 5 times per week, 2 sets of 6 stretches, with each stretch lasting 45 – 90

---

122 Brad J Schoenfeld et al., "Do the Anatomical and Physiological Properties of a Muscle Determine Its Adaptive Response to Different Loading Protocols?," *Physiological Reports* 8, no. 9 (May 2020): e14427–e14427.

123 C. L. Simpson et al., "Stretch Training Induces Unequal Adaptation in Muscle Fascicles and Thickness in Medial and Lateral Gastrocnemii," *Scandinavian Journal of Medicine & Science in Sports* 27, no. 12 (December 2017): 1597–1604.

seconds for 12 weeks, resulted in greater calf muscle fascicle length and cross-sectional area compared to the other calf that was not stretched.[124]

SUMMARY: Calf muscles will grow in response to both light and heavy weight training when sets are taken to near failure or close to failure. Stretching the calf muscles between sets can possibly increase muscle growth.

LIGHT WEIGHT, HIGH REPS ARE TOUGHER

A drawback of using light weight training for muscle growth is that they are more psychologically uncomfortable to perform. When research compared subjects using light weight (25-30 compared to moderate weight (8-12 reps), researchers found that the high reps caused more discomfort, fatigue, and less enjoyment.[125] Using a heavier weight recruits more fast-twitch fibers. Fast-twitch muscle fibers, which are more prone to muscle growth, are activated using heavier weights that allow fewer reps. Using a light weight can still recruit these fast-twitch fibers; it takes longer to activate them, which only occurs when you approach muscular failure. Recently, a study found that full muscle activation can occur by lifting a light weight to failure, similar to using a heavy weight. The drawback is that fatigue may occur before that threshold for type II muscle fiber activation. In contrast, lifting heavy weight causes more muscle fiber activation than lifting a light weight to failure in a shorter time frame.[126] In a study by Morton et al., subjects that trained with light weight to failure had similar

---

124 Joli Panidi et al., "Muscle Architectural and Functional Adaptations Following 12-Weeks of Stretching in Adolescent Female Athletes," *Frontiers in Physiology* 12 (2021): 1088.

125 Alex S. Ribeiro et al., "Acute Effects of Different Training Loads on Affective Responses in Resistance-Trained Men," *International Journal of Sports Medicine* 40, no. 13 (December 2019): 850–55.

126 Tyler W. D. Muddle et al., "Effects of Fatiguing, Submaximal High – versus Low-Torque Isometric Exercise on Motor Unit Recruitment and Firing Behavior," *Physiological Reports* 6, no. 8 (April 2018): e13675.

type I and type II glycogen depletion and increases in key anabolic signaling proteins as those training with a heavier weight. When training with higher or lower loads, when loads are lifted to complete failure, it leads to equivalent muscle hypertrophy and occurs in both type I and type II fibers.[127]

HIGH REPS LEAD TO A DETERIORATION IN FORM

Doing super high reps also leads to a deterioration of exercise form, leading to an increased risk of injury. One study had subjects perform 55 reps of squats. The researchers measured their squat biomechanics and found that the higher repetitions caused by fatigue resulted in a deterioration of the squat form. The study suggests that technique changes in high repetition sets do not favor optimal strength development and may increase the risk of injury, clearly questioning the safety and efficacy of such resistance training programming.[128]

HOW LIGHT IS TOO LIGHT FOR MUSCLE GROWTH

If you don't train to failure or near failure when using a light weight, you won't recruit all the muscle fibers, resulting in less overall tension on the muscle. This was demonstrated in a 2018 study in which subjects trained with different intensities to complete muscular failure with a similar total workload for twelve weeks. Subjects trained with 20%, 40%, 60%, and 80% of their 1-repetition maximum. Training at 40, 60, or 80% of one-repetition maximum 1RM led to similar muscle growth, whereas the 20% of 1RM groups had less biceps and quad growth. This suggests that light

127 Robert W. Morton et al., "Muscle Fibre Activation Is Unaffected by Load and Repetition Duration When Resistance Exercise Is Performed to Task Failure," *The Journal of Physiology* 597, no. 17 (September 2019): 4601–13.

128 David R. Hooper et al., "Effects of Fatigue from Resistance Training on Barbell Back Squat Biomechanics," *Journal of Strength and Conditioning Research* 28, no. 4 (April 2014): 1127–34.

weight will produce suboptimal growth, and weights above 85% won't further increase muscle growth.[129] Thus, using a weight that you can use for more than 30-40 reps will be less conducive for muscle growth than using reps in the 15-30 rep ranges. To reiterate, high repetitions exercises are harder psychologically and much less enjoyable but can produce similar increases to heavier weight.

SUMMARY: You can gain muscle in an extensive range of repetitions. You can gain muscle with 8-10 reps or 20 reps if the sets are taken to near failure (i.e., 2~3 RIR). Researchers have also found similar increases in anabolic signaling pathways (i.e., cellular pathway to stimulate muscle growth) between 2-4 reps and 10-14 reps when completed to failure.[130] It is probably not important to worry about staying in a particular repetition range if the weight is sufficient and repetitions are taken close to exhaustion. Using a weight that is too light (<20% of a 1RM) can cause a good muscle pump but will not increase muscle growth.

MUSCLEGATE: A GOOD MUSCLE PUMP MEANS MUSCLE GROWTH IS OCCURRING

THE TRUTH EXPOSED: The muscle pump is what most lifters strive to achieve in a workout. Arnold Schwarzenegger called it "the greatest feeling you can get in the gym." Whether the muscle pump builds muscle is debatable. There are some lifters that literally "chase the pump." This means people are jumping from program to program to get better pumps. There is evidence that the muscle pump can lead to long-term muscle growth. One study had lifters train with three sets of 80% of a 1-RM and measured

---

129 Thiago Lasevicius et al., "Effects of Different Intensities of Resistance Training with Equated Volume Load on Muscle Strength and Hypertrophy," *European Journal of Sport Science* 18, no. 6 (July 2018): 772–80.

130 Adam M. Gonzalez et al., "Intramuscular Anabolic Signaling and Endocrine Response Following High Volume and High Intensity Resistance Exercise Protocols in Trained Men," *Physiological Reports* 3, no. 7 (July 2015).

muscle thickness or a pumped muscle after exercise. Immediately post-exercise, as expected, the muscle size was larger (8.3%), but after six weeks of training, there was a chronic change in muscle growth by 2.9%. There was a positive relationship between muscle pumps after exercise and increases in muscle growth. This does not mean that muscle pumps cause muscle growth, but it shows a *correlation* between muscle pumps and muscle growth.[131]

Remember that muscle growth can occur anywhere in the 40-60% of a 1-RM range when training to failure, whereas less than 20% results in sub-optimal responses. You can get a good pump using a light weight (i.e., 20% of a 1RM), but as the research suggests, there are minimal increases in muscle growth. Also, keep in mind the study mentioned earlier in the book that muscle growth was similar for lifters using a heavy weight with 3–5 reps and those using 12–15 reps when the total volume was equated. A 3–5 rep protocol is not a great muscle pump protocol, but it still grows muscle. Getting a good muscle pump is not essential for muscle growth, but it is still a great feeling and should not be under-emphasized, as it plays a huge psychological effect. Who does not like feeling the muscle pump?

SARCOPLASMIC HYPERTROPHY

There is some evidence of sarcoplasmic hypertrophy with high volume pump-style training. Sarcoplasmic hypertrophy refers to the fluid in the muscle cell. Sarcoplasm hypertrophy refers to increased fluid and energy resources (ATP, glycogen, creatine phosphate, and water) and sarcoplasmic proteins in the muscle. Thus, sarcoplasmic hypertrophy occurs when *the volume of fluid and other non-contractile proteins in the muscle increase*. This differs from myofibrillar hypertrophy because the muscle itself increases. Think about when you take creatine monohydrate for a few days in large

---

131 Tetsuya Hirono et al., "Relationship Between Muscle Swelling and Hypertrophy Induced by Resistance Training," *Journal of Strength and Conditioning Research*, January 3, 2020.

dosages (i.e., loading phase of 25 grams for 7 days), you will get an increase in muscle size, but it's from the fluid content and not actual changes in the muscle fiber itself.[132]

It's well documented that bodybuilders have much larger fibers than other athletes in other sports. For example, studies have compared muscle biopsies of non-athletes, elite weightlifters, and bodybuilders. The body-builders had the largest muscle fibers (88% larger than the controls and 67% larger than the power athletes).[133] Bodybuilders have bigger muscles, but is it due to sarcoplasmic hypertrophy? In 2019, a study found that when subjects trained with a high volume sarcoplasmic stimulating training (i.e., 1 sets to failure followed by 20 second rest periods with various weight reductions) had greater increases in arm muscle thickness compared to a traditional resistance exercise group (i.e., 8 sets to failure). However, there were no measurements of sarcoplasmic volume.[134] In another study, researchers measured actual changes in the sarcoplasmic fluid by measuring the changes in proteins in the sarcoplasma. Researchers had subjects train three days a week, but they ramped their sets from 10 to 32 sets per week. Fatigue City!! They kept the weight at a relatively light weight at 60% of a 1-RM, consistent with a bodybuilding routine. They also did not train to failure in this study. At the end of the study, shockingly, the high-volume training caused a dilution of muscle fibers because the muscle fibers did not change. Still, there was an increase in sarcoplasmic proteins, which increased in muscle size! So, we have real studies showing that the muscle is getting bigger without increasing actual muscle fibers but an increase

---

132 Michael E. Powers et al., "Creatine Supplementation Increases Total Body Water Without Altering Fluid Distribution," *Journal of Athletic Training* 38, no. 1 (2003): 44–50.

133 J. P. Meijer et al., "Single Muscle Fibre Contractile Properties Differ between Body-Builders, Power Athletes and Control Subjects," *Experimental Physiology* 100, no. 11 (November 2015): 1331–41.

134 Fernando Noronha de Almeida et al., "Acute Effects of the New Method Sarcoplasma Stimulating Training Versus Traditional Resistance Training on Total Training Volume, Lactate and Muscle Thickness," *Frontiers in Physiology* 10 (2019): 579.

in sarcoplasmic expansion.[135] This suggests that low weight, high volume "pump" workouts can increase muscle size through increases in sarcoplasmic proteins but no changes in the actual muscle fiber itself. Another benefit of the study was that the subjects experienced very little muscle damage, despite doing high volume training with light weight. This suggests that high volume, pump-style workouts can lead to increases in size through sarcoplasmic hypertrophy. The jury is still out whether we can say that high-volume exercise leads to genuine changes in sarcoplasmic hypertrophy, but the preliminary evidence is promising.

It's been advocated throughout this book to change sets, reps, contraction velocity, etc., frequently. A recent study compared sarcoplasmic hypertrophy with two different protocols. One protocol performed eight sets of 9-12 reps to failure with 2-minute rest periods (i.e., consistent training protocol). The variable training group workout routine was:

- Variable-weight, eight sets of 25–30 reps to concentric failure/2 min between set rest intervals.

- Variable-sets, 12 sets of 9–12 reps to concentric failure/2 min between set rest intervals.

- Variation in contraction type, eight sets of 10 eccentric contractions at 110% of the load used in the CON leg/2 min between set rest intervals; and

- Variations in rest periods, eight sets of 9–12 reps to concentric failure/4 min between set rest intervals.

At the end of the study, despite both groups gaining muscle mass, only the variable training group resulted in sarcoplasmic hypertrophy. This suggests that instead of using high-rep protocols, one should frequently

---

135 Cody T. Haun et al., "Muscle Fiber Hypertrophy in Response to 6 Weeks of High volume Resistance Training in Trained Young Men Is Largely Attributed to Sarcoplasmic Hypertrophy," PloS one, 14(6), e0215267.

manipulate training stress by changing all the program variables.[136] It should also be emphasized that the frequent manipulation training variable group used a higher training volume than the constant training group. Whether the changes in sarcoplasmic hypertrophy were because of greater volume or frequent manipulation of training variables needs more research to unravel this mystery. This suggests that frequent manipulation of training variables, rather than just performing high rep protocols, can increase size through sarcoplasmic hypertrophy.

MUSCLEGATE: WOMEN NEED TO TRAIN WITH HIGH REPETITIONS TO GAIN MUSCLE.

THE TRUTH EXPOSED: One of the biggest gym myths that won't go away is that women will get bulky if they use heavy weights. The other notorious myth in women's fitness circles is that they just want to "tone" the muscle by light weights. Toning means gaining muscle while losing body fat. First, your diet will determine whether you lose body fat, not your training. Women can gain muscle while losing fat simultaneously while following a high protein diet in conjunction with resistance exercise.[137] Women in this training study used a combination of heavy, moderate, and light weight training comprising five sets of 3-5 repetitions, four sets of 9-11 repetitions, and three sets of 14-16 repetitions. Performing high rep sets while not in a caloric deficit will not decrease body fat. It is more advantageous for women to train with heavier weights. One study found that women gained more muscle when they trained with heavier weight. For six weeks, the study had women train with SuperSlow training (i.e.,

---

136 Carlton D. Fox et al., "Frequent Manipulation of Resistance Training Variables Promotes Myofibrillar Spacing Changes in Resistance-Trained Individuals," *Frontiers in Physiology* 12 (2021): 2239.

137 Bill I. Campbell et al., "Effects of High Versus Low Protein Intake on Body Composition and Maximal Strength in Aspiring Female Physique Athletes Engaging in an 8-Week Resistance Training Program," *International Journal of Sport Nutrition and Exercise Metabolism* 28, no. 6 (November 1, 2018): 580–85.

~40-60% of a 1RM) or a traditional strength training routine (~80-85% of a 1RM) taken to muscular failure. The normal conventional strength training group of women gained more muscle than the SuperSlow group.[138] Again, remember from the previous section that heavy and light weight can promote muscle growth to the same extent if the volume is similar. There are drawbacks to light weight training, as it's more fatiguing to perform and reduces the number of effective reps. It's much more effective for a woman to use a heavier weight because it's more effective for stimulating muscle growth than light weights. The notion that women should use "toning" exercises or high repetitions is flawed because resistance exercise must meet a certain intensity threshold to build muscle; therefore, using a very light weight is not the best approach to achieve the desired stimulus of building muscle while losing body fat.

The fear of gaining bulky muscles is a flawed concept. Most women will see men using heavier weights and believe they achieved their overly muscular appearance by using heavy weights. There are hormonal and genetic differences, but women respond equally to training as men. When men and women are put on resistance training programs, while men make greater absolute gains (total gains) in muscle due to testosterone, relative gains in muscle (i.e., the percentage gains based on their body size) are similar. Women tend to make greater upper body strength gains than men. Relative upper body strength gains were 29% in women compared with 17% in males.[139]

138 Mark D. Schuenke et al., "Early-Phase Muscular Adaptations in Response to Slow-Speed versus Traditional Resistance-Training Regimens," *European Journal of Applied Physiology* 112, no. 10 (October 1, 2012): 3585–95.

139 Brandon M. Roberts, Greg Nuckols, and James W. Krieger, "Sex Differences in Resistance Training: A Systematic Review and Meta-Analysis," *Journal of Strength and Conditioning Research* 34, no. 5 (May 2020): 1448–60.

CHAPTER SUMMARY:

- Using a combination of heavy, moderate, and light weight stimulates muscle growth while giving the joints and ligaments rest.

- Muscle growth can occur from a range of weights lifted from 30% to 85% of a 1RM.

- Training with light weight to stimulate type I muscle growth is highly controversial.

- Light weight training and increased metabolic stress *may* enhance type I muscle growth.

- *SuperSlow* reduces the weight to lift, and lower weight more slowly reduces the effectiveness of your muscle growth.

- Calf muscles can grow in response to both heavy and light weight training.

- High repetitions (>30) can lead to a deterioration in form and are psychologically more difficult.

- It's recommended that for optimal muscle growth, you must use a wide variety of repetition ranges (6-20 repetitions).

- There is a relationship between cell swelling and muscle growth.

- Sarcoplasm hypertrophy with pump-style training *may* occur.

- Sets must be taken close to failure to result in optimal muscle growth.

- Exercise must reach a certain threshold to stimulate muscle growth.

- Light weight training stopping short of failure results in sub-optimal muscle growth.

- Only the last five reps with sufficient intensity are capable of stimulating muscle growth.

- *Junk volume* refers to adding sets but not meeting the minimum expectations for exercise intensity.

- SuperSlow is an example of junk volume because the tension is minimal.

- Heavy weight resistance exercises can increase androgen receptors.

- Repetitions in Reserve are a valuable way of measuring workout fatigue.

- Sets do not need to take sets to complete muscular failure; studies have shown that stopping short of muscular failure results in similar muscle growth.

- There is a relationship between cell swelling and muscle growth.

- Sarcoplasm hypertrophy with pump-style training *may* occur.

CHAPTER 4:

PERIODIZATION

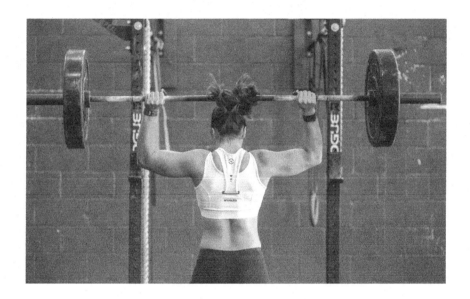

LIFT HEAVY ALL YEAR?

For decades, many bodybuilders have adopted the high-intensity principles of using heavy weight to complete failure with few sets. Keep in mind
that lifting heavier weights (>85% of a 1RM) risks excessive wear and tear
on the joints and predisposes you to injury. A sample of powerlifters found
that 73% were currently injured, and 87% of powerlifters reported having
sustained an injury in the prior year.[140] Ronnie Coleman is one of the greatest bodybuilders ever to compete. His documentary on Netflix is a must-
watch. Ronnie has suffered many injuries and surgeries from all the years of

---

140 Edit Strömbäck et al., ~Prevalence and Consequences of Injuries in Powerlifting:
A Cross-Sectional Study,~ *Orthopaedic Journal of Sports Medicine* 6, no. 5 (May 2018):
2325967118771016.

heavy lifting. Unfortunately, he has had several back surgeries from heavy lifting in the past few years. Remember *that muscle growth can occur from 30% to 85% of a 1RM; you do not have to lift heavy year-round to build muscle.* Using a combination of light, moderate, and heavy weight seems to be a prudent way to train to gain muscle, yet prevent wear and tear on the joints and ligaments. ***Always remember that it's better to use a lighter weight with better technique than to use heavy weight with improper form.*** Using a full range of motion is always optimal for muscle growth. You don't have to lift heavy all year long to build muscle because there are many ways to increase tension on the muscle without using a heavier weight.

PROGRESSIVE OVERLOAD

When most people think of tension overload, they assume to do more exercise! Progressive overload can be defined as meeting or exceeding a necessary physiological stimulus for muscle growth. Most people in the gym just use the assumption of just training harder to build more muscle. ***You can train harder, but it won't always translate into added muscle growth.*** For example, you can train to failure every set, do forced reps, and add more sets, but as you will read later, this can be counterproductive for muscle growth (Chapter 5). This is not the most effective way to train because it does not account for the body's ability to recuperate and fatigue that occurs during and after exercise. The assumption of just doing more is clearly wrong, as studies have found that increasing volume (sets x reps) works up to a certain point; after that, a regression in muscle size occurs. In a meta-analysis published in 2007, the author found that increasing volume (i.e., sets x reps) followed a dose-dependent curve with a greater gain in muscle mass increasing with volume but diminishing returns as volume increases further. It was found that moderate volume (i.e., ~30-60 repetitions per session) yielded the largest response.[141] Progressive overload is the progression in overall stimulus due to *previous adaptations.* Progressive overload allows the progressive adaptations within a single training session. There are designated training blocks for periods of recuperation and fatigue management. The fundamental principle behind progressive overload is the capacity for performance to improve!

Progressive overload is the foundation in which muscles grow; muscles adapt to training; therefore, one must keep overloading the muscle (sets, reps, and weight) to make positive adaptations. We have all heard the story of *Milo of Croton,* who developed strength by carrying a calf on his shoulders each day. As the calf grew bigger, he was able to get progressively stronger until, eventually, he could carry a full-grown bull on his shoulders. As good as this story is, the human body does not respond this way. You do not continuously keep getting stronger and stronger with each workout continuously; if that were the case, we would all be squatting 1000 pounds, but this does not happen. If you tried to add 10 pounds to your squat each day you trained legs, strength gains eventually hit a plateau. You will eventually begin to overtrain, and your progress will regress because the body simply can't adapt to adding weight to each workout without a break. Continuously adding weight to each workout will eventually lead to overtraining. Several biochemical responses occur during overtraining, including increases in cortisol, reduction in testosterone to cortisol ratios, and increased muscle damage, resulting in subsequent reductions in muscle mass and strength. *The single greatest marker of overtraining is a reduction in performance.*

Progressive overload can be accomplished by manipulating training variables, such as weight, sets, reps, increasing workout frequency, etc. There is no definitive answer as to the best way to accomplish progressive overload. You can either add weight and use the same number of reps, use

141 Mathias Wernbom, Jesper Augustsson, and Roland Thomeé, ~The Influence of Frequency, Intensity, Volume and Mode of Strength Training on Whole Muscle Cross-Sectional Area in Humans,~ *Sports Medicine (Auckland, N.Z.)* 37, no. 3 (2007): 225–64.

the same weight for each workout, but do more repetitions, or add sets. The most common weight progression is once you have hit your desired rep range, increase the weight by 5-10%.

COMMON METHODS TO INCREASE PROGRESSIVE OVERLOAD OF MUSCLE

- Increase weight within a rep range

- Increase reps with a given weight

- Increase number of sets

- Increase frequency (increasing total work volume)

- Change exercise technique to increase demand for a given muscle group

- Change repetition tempo

- Add Intensity Techniques (rest-pause, drop sets, supersets)

- Increase the tension on the muscle with mind-muscle connection

PERIODIZATION

In 1945, Dr. Thomas L. DeLorme, an army physician, designed a revolutionary new rehabilitation technique. Instead of using his past recommendations traditional rehabilitation model of 7 sets of 10 repetitions in each exercise, DeLorme's new model recommended was 3 sets of 10. One set was done at 50% of the patient's 10RM, 1 at 75%, and finally 1 at 100% of 10RM. Once a patient could perform >10 repetitions on the final set, the weights were "progressed" accordingly.[142] The brilliance of DeLorme's research was that he paved the foundation of all modern-day strength training programs

---

142 Janice S. Todd, Jason P. Shurley, and Terry C. Todd, "Thomas L. DeLorme and the Science of Progressive Resistance Exercise," *Journal of Strength and Conditioning Research* 26, no. 11 (November 2012): 2913–23.

for increasing strength and hypertrophy. His research was more than just "lifting weights" but the ability to provide a resistance training program that improved physical performance. There are basic training principles for increasing strength and muscle hypertrophy.[143]

- Progressive overload: The workout stimulus must gradually increase over time to further improve performance.

- Specificity: The training adaptations are specific to the stimulus applied.

- Variation (and/or Periodization): Appropriate training volume and intensity manipulation, speed of movement, and exercise selection.

- Individuality: The magnitude of the adaptation to the training stimulus (i.e., performance improvement) is different for each person.

Periodization has various blocks or cycles that are classified by amounts of time: macro (annual), meso (weeks to months), and micro (days to weekly). Over the course of a training cycle, the tension on the muscle is gradually increased (weight, reps, sets). If the training response is too strong and the body cannot recuperate, this leads to overtraining, a maladaptive response in which the body regresses.

Overtraining results in a sustained decrease in performance for months. Many lifters like to say that they are overtraining if they have not made progress, but a true physiological overtraining response is very difficult to induce. In a 2020 systematic review of overtraining research in resistance training, 10 of the 22 studies where researchers attempted to induce overreaching or overtraining, they failed, as no reduction in performance

---

143 Michael Stone, Steven Plisk, and David Collins, "Strength and Conditioning," *Sports Biomechanics* 1, no. 1 (January 1, 2002): 79–103.

was observed.[144] There are genuine cases of overtraining; for example, the legendary study by Fry and colleagues would break any lifter. Participants performed 10 sets of singles with a 1RM with 2-minute rest periods for two weeks during the study. Let me repeat that: "They did 10 max squat tests twice per week!" After that, their 1RM performance dropped by 26.8 pounds.[145] The subjects had reduced nerve stimulation, increased markers of muscle damage (i.e., creatine kinase), and decreased lactate responses during exercise. Overtraining can occur; it rarely occurs with a typical lifter who goes to the gym a few days a week. Overtraining is much more likely to occur in endurance athletes than in strength athletes.[146]

There is also a term called *overreaching*, meaning a person's physiological stress is taken above a person's limit. A deload or break is immediately taken, followed by a growth and recovery phase. There is a difference between overreaching and overtraining. Overreaching is a planned escalation of physiological stress, followed by fatigue management and recovery. Overtraining is the continued inability to adapt to a training demand, with a subsequent reduction in performance. A proper training program should have periods of overreaching to enhance adaptations, but never to the point of overtraining. After overreaching, deloads, in which the total training volume and intensity are reduced, should be performed every 4-8 weeks. Deloads are necessary for both physical and psychological breaks from strenuous exercise (i.e., discussed in Chapter 8). There are several periodization models to increase tension overload, such as linear, non-linear, and reverse linear.

---

144 Clementine Grandou et al., "Overtraining in Resistance Exercise: An Exploratory Systematic Review and Methodological Appraisal of the Literature," *Sports Medicine* 50, no. 4 (April 2020): 815–28.

145 A. C. Fry et al., "Performance Decrements with High-Intensity Resistance Exercise Overtraining," *Medicine and Science in Sports and Exercise* 26, no. 9 (September 1994): 1165–73.

146 Christopher M. Norris, Overtraining Syndrome – an Overview. Managing Sports Injuries (Fourth Edition), Churchill Livingstone, 2011,Pages 59-83.

LINEAR PERIODIZATION

Linear periodization is the most popular method of training. This form of periodization involves increasing intensity (i.e., weight) and decreasing volume (i.e., sets and reps) throughout multiple mesocycles in an annual training plan.

EXAMPLE OF A LINEAR PERIODIZATION PROGRAM:

Week 1: 3 Sets X 10 Repetitions @ 70% of a 1RM

Week 2: 3 Sets X 8 Repetitions @ 75% of a 1RM

Week 3: 3 Sets X 6 Repetitions @ 80% of a 1RM

Week 4: 3 Sets X 5 Repetitions @ 85% of a 1RM

*Weight or intensity is gradually increasing while volume is decreasing.

NON-LINEAR OR UNDULATING PERIODIZATION

Non-Linear Periodization involves constantly changing various components such as the weight, sets, and reps during the cycle. Non-linear periodization changes multiple variables like exercises, volume, intensity, rest period, and training adaptation frequently. This is in direct contrast to a linear periodization program that focuses on the gradual increase of one variable. The theory behind this type of training is that alternating heavy and light days allows muscle fibers, joints, and connective tissue to recuperate on light days while maintaining muscle tension. Undulating periodization can be broken down into daily undulating and weekly undulating periodization.

EXAMPLE OF A NON-LINEAR PERIODIZATION:

Week 1-2: Hypertrophy 5 sets X 8-12 RM, 1-minute rest periods

Week 3-4: Strength, 4 sets X 4-8 reps RM, 3–5-minute rest periods

Week 5-6: Power, 4 sets X 2-3 RM, 3–5-minute rest periods

*Use a combination of all the training variables (sets, reps, weight, rest periods).

REVERSE PERIODIZATION

Reverse periodization is like linear periodization but in reverse; each macrocycle starts with heavier weights at the beginning and less volume (sets and reps) and progresses to lighter weights and more volume (more sets and reps).

EXAMPLE OF A REVERSE PERIODIZATION:

Week 1: 3 Sets X 5 Repetitions @ % 85 of a 1RM

Week 2: 3 Sets X 6 Repetitions @ % 80 of a 1RM

Week 3: 3 Sets X 8 Repetitions @ % 75 of a 1RM

Week 4: 3 Sets X 10 Repetitions @ % 70 of a 1RM

*Weight is progressively decreasing as the volume increases.

All these principles involve modifying one or more training variables. The goal of periodization is to improve performance and for people reading this book to gain muscle and reduce the risk of overtraining.

The research suggests that both linear and undulating periodization are equally effective for muscle growth.[147,148] However, one study

---

147 J. Grgic et al., "Should Resistance Training Programs Aimed at Muscular Hypertrophy Be Periodized? A Systematic Review of Periodized versus Non-Periodized Approaches," *Science & Sports* 33, no. 3 (June 1, 2018): e97–104.

148 Jozo Grgic et al., "Effects of Linear and Daily Undulating Periodized Resistance Training Programs on Measures of Muscle Hypertrophy: A Systematic Review and Meta-Analysis," *PeerJ* 5 (2017): e3695.

found reverse periodization to be less effective than linear periodization for muscle growth. Researchers had subjects assigned to either a linear periodization routine (i.e., light weight progresses to heavy weight) or reverse linear periodization (heavy weight progresses to less weight and higher reps). The researchers reported that those that performed linear periodization or gradually increased the weight over a period resulted in a seven-pound increase in lean mass. In contrast, the reverse periodization group decreased weight and gained only three pounds.[149] Contrary to the previous study's findings, Camargo et al. found that training blocks of strength phases preceding a hypertrophy phase or vice versa resulted in a similar increase in lean muscle mass and strength. Resistance-trained men were randomized into two groups. One group completed six weeks of hypertrophy training, followed by six weeks of strength training. The other group completed the same blocks of training in the opposite order. Both groups used the same volume over the six-week training study. The strength block trained with compound exercises in the 2-4 RM range. The hypertrophy block trained with compound and single-joint exercises performed in the 10-12 RM range. At the end of the study, both groups had similar increases in muscle strength and muscle mass when the volume was similar.[150] Remember what I said earlier about jumping to conclusions with one research study? The two studies above are perfect examples of conflicting study results.

There seems to be a minor advantage in alternating sets and reps over a mesocycle. One study compared a non-periodized (kept the same volume), a traditional periodization, and an undulating periodization program for 12 weeks. The non-periodized group performed 3 sets of an 8 RM for 12 weeks. The traditional periodized group alternated both sets

---

149 Jonato Prestes et al., "Comparison of Linear and Reverse Linear Periodization Effects on Maximal Strength and Body Composition," *The Journal of Strength & Conditioning Research* 23, no. 1 (2009).

150 Júlio Benvenutti Bueno DE Camargo et al., ~Order of Resistance Training Cycles to Develop Strength and Muscle Thickness in Resistance-Trained Men: A Pilot Study,~ *International Journal of Exercise Science* 14, no. 4 (2021): 644–56.

and reps every few weeks. The undulating program alternated sets and reps on a weekly basis. The total sets and reps were equated between the groups, so the total workload was similar, whereas training intensity was manipulated throughout the study. Leg muscle size increased in all groups non-periodized (8.1%), traditional periodization (11.3%), and undulating periodization (8.7%). In the first six weeks, all groups increased muscle size; however, *only the conventional periodization and undulating periodization group increased leg muscle size from weeks 6-12.*[151] There was a slight advantage in the magnitude of muscle growth for the periodized groups over the non-periodized. This suggests that volume is a key factor for muscle growth; however, there is an advantage in changing both sets and reps throughout a training cycle.

It's important to emphasize when the volume (sets x reps) and intensity (% of a 1RM) are similar; it does not matter whether you change these variables daily or weekly. For example, when researchers compared subjects who used a daily combination of different intensities and rep ranges (i.e., combined heavy and light training each workout) compared to a weekly undulating program (used the same rep range for the entire week, then changing rep and set schemes the next week). *At the end of the study, similar increases in muscle occurred between both groups, provided the total volume and intensity were similar.*[152] This suggests that people looking to gain muscle need to strategically periodize their workouts by changing both volume and intensity for optimal muscle growth. It does not seem to matter whether the changes in reps and sets are done daily or weekly.

---

151 Eduardo O. De Souza et al., "Different Patterns in Muscular Strength and Hypertrophy Adaptations in Untrained Individuals Undergoing Nonperiodized and Periodized Strength Regimens," *Journal of Strength and Conditioning Research* 32, no. 5 (May 2018): 1238–44.

152 Markus Antretter et al., "The Hatfield-System versus the Weekly Undulating Periodised Resistance Training in Trained Males," *International Journal of Sports Science & Coaching* 13, no. 1 (February 1, 2018): 95–103.

HAVE A PLAN. USE A JOURNAL

It always amazes me that when I go to the gym, I have a specific workout in which I am actively manipulating my sets, reps, and weight to achieve a greater workout stimulus. I look around, and rarely do I see anyone tracking their workout with notebooks or phone apps. One of the biggest mistakes earlier in my training was I never kept a training journal or tracked volume and intensity. How do you expect to grow if you are not tracking your workouts? Can you imagine a track and field coach without a stopwatch gauging an athlete's performance? If you don't have a plan, do not expect to succeed in gaining muscle. Six-Time Mr. Olympia Dorian Yates kept a detailed training journal for how he trained, what he ate, how he felt during his workouts, mood, etc. Dorian didn't believe in prep coaches because he knew his body better than anyone. He kept meticulous notes on his calories, training reps, volume, weight lifted, etc. How can you track progress in the gym without keeping a training journal? It's like conducting a lab experiment and not recording your notes and results.

You should track your weight and take girth measurements regularly. Using a simple tape circumference is accurate and is comparable to ultrasound for measuring lean mass.[153] Take regular measurements of your chest, calves, thighs, arms, waist, hips, etc., while also tracking body weight with a scale. You can use various electric scales that measure lean muscle mass and fat mass but keep in mind that they have a higher degree of error. A study comparing various electric scales found that fat mass, absolute errors ranged from –2.2 kg to –4.4 kg (1 to 2 pounds) and muscular mass, absolute errors were + 4.0 kg to – 6.6 kg (1.8 to – 3 pounds).[154] You are much better off using a regular skinfold for accuracy. Also, it's important to

---

153 Kieran O'Sullivan, David Sainsbury, and Richard O'Connor, "Measurement of Thigh Muscle Size Using Tape or Ultrasound Is a Poor Indicator of Thigh Muscle Strength," *Isokinetics and Exercise Science* 17 (August 26, 2009): 145–53.

154 Justine Frija-Masson et al., "Accuracy of Smart Scales on Weight and Body Composition: Observational Study," *JMIR MHealth and UHealth* 9, no. 4 (April 30, 2021): e22487.

take regular weight measurements to determine if you are gaining weight in conjunction with progress photos every 4-8 weeks.

One of the key motivating factors to write this book was all the time, money, and progress that I lost on supplements, program hopping, and not tracking my workouts. The most valuable thing I could have done was hire a coach or use a workout template designed by experts to increase muscle growth. I would highly recommend going to an evidence-based bodybuilding website with experts specializing in muscle growth, such as:

- Renaissance Training:
  https://renaissanceperiodization.com/rp-store

- JPS Health and Fitness:
  https://www.jpshealthandfitness.com.au/product/
  free-jps-home-workout-template/

- Dr. Muscle Workout App: https://dr-muscle.com/

- Revive Stronger Coaching:
  https://revivestronger.com/online-coaching/

- Muscle and Strength Pyramids:
  https://muscleandstrengthpyramids.com/

- 3D Muscle Journey:
  https://3dmusclejourney.com/

These are amazing resources for having a coach assist you with your training program. They have workout templates to download and online coaches and resources for a science-based workout.

CHAPTER SUMMARY:

- Progressive overload can be accomplished by manipulating training variables such as weight, sets, reps, less rest periods between sets, increasing workout frequency, etc.

- When volume or total workload is similar, there is no difference in which form of periodization you perform.

- Keeping a training journal is a valuable way to track progressive overload.

CHAPTER 5:

THE OPTIMAL NUMBER OF SETS FOR MUSCLE GROWTH

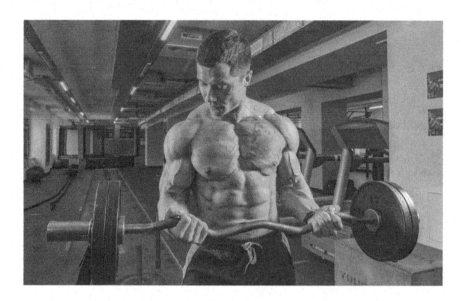

TRAINING VOLUME (SETS X REPS)

When classifying how much work has been performed over time, research-ers often use what is called *volume*. The volume of a workout is commonly referred to as the number of *sets x reps* you perform; however, the amount of weight you lift also affects the volume. The time taken to complete the exercise will also affect the volume. Most lifters will count sets and reps, but few people will measure the workout set's duration (time taken to complete the set). There are many ways to measure training volume, but for gaining muscle, focus on the total training volume, which is the *total amount of weight lifted over a period.* Volume can be measured in multiple ways, but for gaining muscle, three crucial factors are essential for stimulating muscle growth:

- The sets must be sufficient in volume to stimulate muscle growth.

- The sets must be of adequate intensity to stimulate muscle growth.

- The sets must be taken to a proximity to muscular failure (i.e., not to complete failure, but close to failure).

Two workouts can simplify the relationship between volume, tension, and muscle growth. A.) Is a classic bodybuilding program, B.) Is a traditional powerlifting program.

1. 3 sets x 10 reps x 225 (weight on the bar) =total workout volume 6,750

2. 3 sets x 5 reps x 315 (weight on the bar) =total workout volume 4,725

Workout A has a greater potential for muscle growth because it results in a greater workout volume. Now, if the powerlifter in Workout B increased his sets to 4, his workout volume would go up to 6,300, and the chances of muscle growth are much greater to the bodybuilding protocol because his volume is now higher. When researchers compared a bodybuilding workout (i.e., 4 sets of 8-12 reps to failure) to a max strength testing group (i.e., 5 sets with a 1 RM), the bodybuilding group gained more muscle. However, the bodybuilding group performed more volume (sets x reps), resulting in larger increases in muscle growth.[155] Studies have shown that *muscle growth is identical when workout volume is equated* or similar between

---

155 Kevin T. Mattocks et al., "Practicing the Test Produces Strength Equivalent to Higher Volume Training," *Medicine and Science in Sports and Exercise* 49, no. 9 (September 2017): 1945–54.

powerlifting and bodybuilding style workouts. As you will learn later in the chapters, volume is related to muscle growth up to a certain point; thereafter, too much volume is counterproductive for muscle growth.

As you will see with numerous research studies in this book, doing more sets does not always lead to greater muscle growth. The increase in volume that you can tolerate in a training cycle depends on the current training volume one is using. For example, it's much easier for a person who is training with 10 sets per bodypart per week to increase to 12 sets compared to a person using 3 sets per body part per week. When trying to increase volume, it's easier to add sets rather than increase the weight of each workout. With strength training, frequent and monotonous training performed at high intensity seems to be the variable that most often leads to overtraining.[156] This suggests that periods of heavy lifting (i.e., high-intensity exercise) for a sustained period can lead to systemic fatigue and overtraining syndrome.

Most lifters keep thinking the amount of weight lifted is the most critical driver of muscle growth; *the volume of sets is a better driver of muscle growth than the amount of weight used when exercise intensity is sufficiently high, up to a certain point.* A study found that when subjects increased their volume by an average of ~20% compared to their previous *self-reported volume* resulted in greater muscle growth.[157] However, there is a point in which adding more sets will no longer contribute to muscle growth; it's an individual adaptation process.

Muscles grow by escalating the overall tension placed on the muscle, which can be accomplished by modifying any of these variables. One must ask how much additional total workload I can put on my body

---

156 Clementine Grandou et al., "Overtraining in Resistance Exercise: An Exploratory Systematic Review and Methodological Appraisal of the Literature," *Sports Medicine* 50, no. 4 (April 2020): 815–28.

157 Maíra C. Scarpelli et al., ~Muscle Hypertrophy Response Is Affected by Previous Resistance Training Volume in Trained Individuals.,~ *Journal of Strength and Conditioning Research*, February 27, 2020.

without fatiguing it to the point when you can no longer recuperate from your workouts. Dr. Mike Israetel has termed maximum recoverable volume as the highest training volume an athlete can do during the training cycle and *still recover*. I would highly recommend reading his book, *"How Much Should I Train?" An Introduction to Training Volume Landmarks*.[158] It should be mentioned that there is a direct relationship between training volume (sets) and muscle growth up to a certain point; however, further increases in volume will cause diminishing returns.

Strength loss is a valuable tool to assess performance and muscle damage.[159] As mentioned in the previous chapter, *of all the markers of overtraining you can monitor, a decrease in performance is the most accurate indicator of overtraining*. If your strength is not progressing with each workout, this could indicate that your muscles or nervous system have not yet recuperated between workouts. A week-to-week progression of muscle overload is one of the predominant forms of increasing muscle growth. A person seeking to use a structured, progressive overload resistance training program may wonder: Should I add more weight to the bar each week, add more repetitions, or add sets to provide the best hypertrophy-specific overload? I would highly recommend the article by Dr. Israetel in which he discusses the pros and cons of volume and intensity for hypertrophy titled, *"Mesocycle Progression in Hypertrophy: Volume Versus Intensity."* In sum, Dr. Israetel concludes, ***"Based on the current literature, the likely answer is "some of all 3 (sets, reps, and weight)," but with a progression in set numbers (volume) probably being the most well supported.***[160] It's

---

158 Amazon.Com: "How Much Should I Train?: An Introduction to the Volume Landmarks (Renaissance Periodization Book 5)" EBook: Israetel, Dr. Mike, Hoffmann, Dr. James: Kindle Store.

159 Robert D. Hyldahl and Monica J. Hubal, "Lengthening Our Perspective: Morphological, Cellular, and Molecular Responses to Eccentric Exercise," *Muscle & Nerve* 49, no. 2 (February 2014): 155–70.

160 Mike Israetel et al., "Mesocycle Progression in Hypertrophy: Volume Versus Intensity," *Strength & Conditioning Journal* 42, no. 5 (2020).

suggested that you combine a wide variety of sets, reps, and weight to maximize muscle growth.

POWER-BODYBUILDING FOR MORE MUSCLE GROWTH?

For decades, bodybuilders were told to stay in the 8-10 rep range for muscle growth; however, adding a strength cycle *may boost muscle growth*. It has been suggested that using a combination of light, moderate, and heavy weight produces superior increases in muscle growth. A great example of why bodybuilders should add some strength phases to their workout was a 2020 study. Subjects were assigned to either a combination of strength and bodybuilding training or bodybuilding training alone for eight weeks. The strength and bodybuilding training group performed three weeks of strength training using 1-3 reps for three weeks, then switched to a bodybuilding-style program in which they trained with 8-12 repetitions. The other group used a bodybuilding-style program for eight weeks (8-12 reps). *At the end of the study, the strength and bodybuilding group gained more muscle than the bodybuilding group.*[161] This study is unique because traditionally, one to three reps is considered strength training. Most bodybuilders would never think of incorporating low rep training into their routine, yet this may have the capacity to build more muscle. Again, this is *one* study. More studies replicating this study need to be conducted to duplicate these results to confirm its validity. Still, it suggests that a wide range of stimuli, including heavy and light weight, with a range of various repetitions, may be optimal for increasing muscle. I personally would not recommend singles and doubles for bodybuilding. The risk associated with this type of training is too high for injury. I would recommend a 5-7 rep range for the strength phase. The addition of the strength phase with the

---

161 Leonardo Carvalho et al., "Is Stronger Better? Influence of a Strength Phase Followed by a Hypertrophy Phase on Muscular Adaptations in Resistance-Trained Men," *Research in Sports Medicine (Print)* 29, no. 6 (December 2021): 536–46.

heavier weights may have increased more fast-twitch fiber types, which have the most muscle growth potential, but whether rep ranges can affect fiber types is very controversial. *If building muscle is your primary goal, a majority of your training should be spent in bodybuilding-style workouts; adding a strength phase can result in greater strength gains.* If you are stronger, then technically, you should be able to handle a greater weight (more tension) once you switch back to your bodybuilding protocol. To further emphasize the importance of changing repetitions, an earlier study by the same author found that lifters who varied with weight and rep ranges grew more than those that just used 10-12 reps. In this study, subjects either used a constant 8-12 RM three days a week or a varied protocol that consisted of 2-4 RM on Day 1, 8-12 RM on day 2, and 20-30 RM on Day 3. The varied group tended to have greater increases in muscle size compared to the constant group.[162]

SAMPLE WORKOUT FROM STRENGTH/ HYPERTROPHY STUDY:

Strength Training Weeks	1-3	4 Sets × 1-3 RM
Hypertrophy Training Weeks	4-8	4 Sets × 8-12 RM

THE OPTIMAL NUMBER OF SETS FOR MUSCLE GROWTH

Many scientific scholars debate the optimal number of sets to perform for each body part for maximal muscle growth. In the early '80s, pioneer Mike Mentzer adopted the High-Intensity Training (HIT) philosophy of Arthur Jones and created the *Heavy-Duty Training System.* Both Jones and

---

162 B. J. Schoenfeld et al., "Effects of Varied Versus Constant Loading Zones on Muscular Adaptations in Trained Men," *International Journal of Sports Medicine* 37, no. 6 (June 2016): 442–47.

Mentzer advocated one to two sets to complete muscular failure. Anything beyond this was considered overtraining. Contrary to this training, other bodybuilders like Arnold Schwarzenegger advocated more than 20+ sets per body part. This section will take on some of the most common myths regarding low and high volume and its influence on muscle growth.

MUSCLEGATE: 1 SET OF HIGH INTENSITY EXERCISE TO FAILURE IS ALL YOU NEED FOR MUSCLE GROWTH

THE TRUTH EXPOSED: You can grow with as little as one set per body part *if you are a beginner*. If you are an intermediate or advanced lifter, you will need more sets. A lifter will gradually need to increase the number of sets in their training cycle to keep making gains in muscle growth. Increased volume seems to be especially important for advanced lifters. The body becomes remarkably adaptive to resistance exercise; a higher exercise stimulus threshold will be needed for muscle growth. Multiple sets increase muscle protein synthesis and anabolic signaling pathways in muscle. Studies have found a positive correlation between volume (i.e., sets) and muscle protein synthesis.[163,164] Similar to protein synthesis, anabolic signaling pathways are increased after multiple sets compared to single sets.[165] For example, one study found that 10 sets of 10 reps resulted in a greater muscle anabolic signaling pathway activation than 5 sets of 10

163 Vinod Kumar et al., "Muscle Protein Synthetic Responses to Exercise: Effects of Age, Volume, and Intensity," *The Journals of Gerontology. Series A, Biological Sciences and Medical Sciences* 67, no. 11 (November 2012): 1170–77.

164 Felipe Damas et al., "Myofibrillar Protein Synthesis and Muscle Hypertrophy Individualized Responses to Systematically Changing Resistance Training Variables in Trained Young Men," *Journal of Applied Physiology (Bethesda, Md.: 1985)* 127, no. 3 (September 1, 2019): 806–15.

165 Gerasimos Terzis et al., "The Degree of P70 S6k and S6 Phosphorylation in Human Skeletal Muscle in Response to Resistance Exercise Depends on the Training Volume," *European Journal of Applied Physiology* 110, no. 4 (November 2010): 835–43.

reps.[166] Don't misinterpret this study to think that you should start doing 10 sets per exercise. It's a single study showing a greater increase in signaling pathways with more sets. In sum, the greater increases in anabolic signaling pathways and protein synthesis with higher sets can lead to greater muscle growth than single sets.

THE RELATIONSHIP BETWEEN SETS AND MUSCLE GROWTH

The principles of the relationship between volume and increased muscle growth are well documented in Olympic weightlifters. Although weightlifters are interested in peak force development, they often perform hypertrophy cycles. When Olympic lifters go through hypertrophy cycles (3 sets of 10 repetitions), in which volume is highest, there is an increase in muscle size, whereas when they transition to power/strength cycles (3 sets of 5 repetitions) and volume is the lowest results in a decrease in muscle size.[167] Previous studies have found that one set can increase muscle growth. However, muscle growth follows a dose-response curve with moderate (3 sets) and high (5 sets), resulting in greater muscle growth.[168] Baseline levels of muscle mass predicted beneficial responses to higher volume training.[169] This suggests that trained athletes need a greater set/rep stimulus than novice lifters. Multiple sets are superior to a single set

166 Juha P. Ahtiainen et al., "Exercise Type and Volume Alter Signaling Pathways Regulating Skeletal Muscle Glucose Uptake and Protein Synthesis," *European Journal of Applied Physiology* 115, no. 9 (September 2015): 1835–45.

167 Dylan G. Suarez et al., "Phase-Specific Changes in Rate of Force Development and Muscle Morphology Throughout a Block Periodized Training Cycle in Weightlifters," *Sports (Basel, Switzerland)* 7, no. 6 (May 28, 2019): E129.

168 Brad J. Schoenfeld et al., "Resistance Training Volume Enhances Muscle Hypertrophy but Not Strength in Trained Men," *Medicine and Science in Sports and Exercise* 51, no. 1 (January 2019): 94–103.

169 Daniel Hammarström et al., ~Benefits of Higher Resistance-Training Volume Are Related to Ribosome Biogenesis," *The Journal of Physiology* 598, no. 3 (2020): 543–65.

for strength gains, muscle endurance, and arm growth.[170] One of the most compelling arguments for multiple sets for enhancing muscle growth is a meta-analysis by James Krieger, in which he found that muscle growth was the greatest in those that did 2-3 sets versus 1 set. He also found that the 4-6 sets had a slightly better increase in muscle growth than the 2-3 sets. The meta-analysis showed that doing more sets leads to more muscle growth than a single set.[171] The same author later conducted another meta-analysis and reported a linear relationship between sets and muscle growth. Less than 5 sets per week resulted in the least muscle growth (5.4%), whereas more sets, 5-9 sets (6.6%), and 10+ sets (9.8%) resulted in greater increases in lean muscle mass.[172] Other studies have shown that 15 sets per week resulted in greater muscle mass than 9 sets per week.[173] *Based on the research, between 10-20 sets seems to be the threshold for the maximum number of sets per week for muscle growth*. Dr. Schoenfeld, one of the leading experts in muscle growth, was quoted as saying, "10+ sets per week is necessary to maximize the hypertrophic response to resistance exercise. Again, this represents a *minimum threshold.* We now need to determine the maximum upper threshold for volume lies to promote the greatest increases in muscular gains."

On average, probably 3-4 sets per exercise are a suitable target, with 2-4 exercises per body part. In his book *Scientific Principles of Hypertrophy Training,* Dr. Israel recommends that 70% of your volume come from the big compound movements (i.e., multi-joint exercises such as bench press,

---

170 Regis Radaelli et al., "Dose-Response of 1, 3, and 5 Sets of Resistance Exercise on Strength, Local Muscular Endurance, and Hypertrophy," *Journal of Strength and Conditioning Research* 29, no. 5 (May 2015): 1349–58.

171 James W. Krieger, "Single vs. Multiple Sets of Resistance Exercise for Muscle Hypertrophy: A Meta-Analysis," *Journal of Strength and Conditioning Research* 24, no. 4 (April 2010): 1150–59.

172 Brad J. Schoenfeld, Dan Ogborn, and James W. Krieger, "Dose-Response Relationship between Weekly Resistance Training Volume and Increases in Muscle Mass: A Systematic Review and Meta-Analysis," *Journal of Sports Sciences* 35, no. 11 (June 2017): 1073–82.

173 Regis Radaelli et al., "Dose-Response of 1, 3, and 5 Sets of Resistance Exercise on Strength, Local Muscular Endurance, and Hypertrophy," *The Journal of Strength & Conditioning Research* 29, no. 5 (May 2015): 1349–58.

squats, etc.), leaving 30% for isolation work (i.e., leg extensions, leg curls). It's best to use a wide variety of rep ranges for compound and isolation exercises. Compound exercises are more suited to lower reps and isolation exercises to higher reps. Performing high repetitions (>20 reps) with compound movements such as the squat, deadlift, and bench press results in extreme central nervous system and peripheral fatigue. It's no coincidence that you can perform 20 reps of calf raises and feel perfectly fine a minute later, but try 20 reps of squats, and you will be gasping for air. Also, exercise form is less likely to break down with isolation exercises, whereas compound movements have a greater risk of injury with deteriorating exercise form.

FINDING THE RIGHT NUMBER OF SETS THAT WORK FOR YOU

It's well documented that resistance exercise with multiple sets can increase muscle protein synthesis, which stimulates a cascade of events leading to increases in muscle growth.[174,175] There is no universal set range that will work for everyone; for optimal results, some people will need more sets, whereas others will need less. Many people perform too many sets, leading to an imbalanced stimulus to fatigue ratio. The situation can be further worsened if the sets are performed to failure. An increase in training volume results in more muscle damage and greater recuperation time between workouts. A 2019 study had subjects perform either 8 or 12 sets per workout to complete muscular failure. The group that performed 12 sets had a *slightly greater* increase in muscle protein synthesis, but the author suspected this might have been caused due to greater muscle damage for

---

174 K. D. Tipton and R. R. Wolfe, "Exercise, Protein Metabolism, and Muscle Growth," *International Journal of Sport Nutrition and Exercise Metabolism* 11, no. 1 (March 2001): 109–32.

175 S. M. Phillips et al., "Mixed Muscle Protein Synthesis and Breakdown after Resistance Exercise in Humans," *The American Journal of Physiology* 273, no. 1 Pt 1 (July 1997): E99-107.

the 12-set group. *Interestingly, both groups had similar increases in muscle growth.*[176]

When starting a new exercise movement, it's important to start with a few sets and increase the sets as the weeks progress. Unaccustomed exercise is associated with the largest increase in muscle damage in the early phases of training, but this is not associated with muscle growth. Furthermore, increases in muscle growth occur in the later stages of training when muscle damage has been attenuated.[177] Keep in mind that muscle damage is separate from muscle growth. If you constantly damage a muscle, you won't grow muscle; you will lose muscle! A study in powerlifters found evidence of excess muscle damage and disrupted regenerative processes in the muscle. The study's author concluded that the normal regenerative process is most likely disturbed by continuous training with repeated high mechanical stress on the muscles in powerlifters.[178] The key to finding the optimal number of sets to perform is to experiment with increasing sets until fatigue occurs, followed by a subsequent decrease in volume. Unfortunately, there is no magic number of sets that work best for everyone, but 10 sets per bodypart per week is a good starting point based on the research. This can easily be achieved by breaking up your weekly training split so that each body part is trained twice per week. For example, 2-3 sets of incline bench press and pec flyes on Monday and 2-3 sets of bench press and cable cross-over on Thursday.

---

176 Felipe Damas et al., "Resistance Training-Induced Changes in Integrated Myofibrillar Protein Synthesis Are Related to Hypertrophy Only after Attenuation of Muscle Damage," *The Journal of Physiology* 594, no. 18 (September 15, 2016): 5209–22.

177 Giselle Keefe and Craig Wright, "An Intricate Balance of Muscle Damage and Protein Synthesis: The Key Players in Skeletal Muscle Hypertrophy Following Resistance Training," *The Journal of Physiology* 594, no. 24 (December 15, 2016): 7157–58.

178 Anders Eriksson et al., "Hypertrophic Muscle Fibers with Fissures in Power-Lifters; Fiber Splitting or Defect Regeneration?," *Histochemistry and Cell Biology* 126, no. 4 (October 2006): 409–17.

WHEN DO YOU NEED TO ADD SETS?

There is intense debate about how many sets you should add when planning your workout. Some experts believe that if you make progress and get stronger each week, there is no need to add additional sets. Some experts believe that you can increase progressive overload by either increasing the weight or doing more reps while keeping sets the same. In the book *The Muscle and Strength Pyramids*[179], Eric Helms Ph.D. recommends a series of questions that can decide when to add sets.

Has your workout plateaued? If it has not, stick to your current workout routine.

- If your workouts have plateaued, make sure that you are:

    i.   Getting adequate sleep

    ii. Diet is on track with sufficient calories

    iii. Are you training with a minimum of 10 sets per week per body part?

    iv. Are you training with a sufficient intensity level?

    v.   Are you training each body part twice per week?

    vi. Are you recuperating between workouts?

        1. Do you feel tired all the time?

        2. Do you lack the motivation to train?

        3. Are your life stresses in check, or are there circumstances occurring that are causing you stress?

---

179 "The Muscle and Strength Pyramid: Training: Helms, Eric Russell, Morgan, Andy, Valdez, Andrea Marie: 9781090912824: Amazon.Com: Books,"

If you have not addressed these issues, fix these issues first before adding more sets. This book is essential for any serious trainer who wants to understand the fundamentals of volume, intensity, and other training factors required for muscle growth.

Adding sets is warranted if you track your body composition (lean mass) and do not gain muscle. Remember that adding sets should be the last option only when all other training variables have been addressed. If you are progressing in your repetitions or your strength is slowly increasing, there is no need to add sets. Keep in mind that your ability to recuperate from a workout takes longer by adding sets. Adding sets also increases the duration of the time spent in the gym. Before increasing your workout volume, make sure you are hitting your other critical variables for muscle growth, including proper nutrition and sleep, how close you are training to failure, proper exercise form, frequency, etc. Adding another set is best used for lagging body parts. If you have great legs, but your calves are lagging, add additional sets to bring up lagging body parts. If you add sets for every body part, this will lead to a larger increase in systemic fatigue. The *Revive Stronger* website uses the analogy of adding too many sets, and its relationship to fatigue is like comparing the nervous system to an iPhone battery. Each time you open a new app on your phone, it runs in the background and drains the battery faster. Similarly, adding sets for every body part will lead to a larger strain on the nervous system and greater recovery. Start by adding 1 or 2 sets for a single exercise. Make sure you monitor your recovery. If you feel sore or your strength is noticeably dropping, you need more recuperation time between workouts or a decrease in the number of sets. I recommend visiting Dr. Mike Israel's site for more information about volume training: https://renaissanceperiodization.com/.

ARE YOU EATING ENOUGH FOR MORE MUSCLE GROWTH?

Most lifters add volume before checking to ensure other lifestyle factors are in check. You may simply need more calories to grow or are not getting adequate sleep, which is hindering your progress. It is recommended that a calorie surplus of 200-500 calories per day (10-25% caloric surplus) to increase lean mass. Many lifters exceed this amount while attempting to gain muscle mass, but they risk gaining body fat as well. A study in bodybuilders found that bodybuilders consuming a high-calorie diet (6,087 calories per day) gained more muscle, but also more body fat compared to a moderate calorie surplus (4,501 calories per day) who gained less muscle, but also less body fat.[180] The moderate caloric surplus had a 1.5% increase in muscle and a 2.5% increase in fat after 4 weeks. In contrast, the high-calorie surplus gained 3% muscle and 12.4% fat. In most cases, liquid calories in a shake are an easy way to boost calories and protein. It's much easier to consume liquid calories as opposed to whole foods. Mega mass 2,000 calorie shakes, and other high-calorie shakes are unnecessary unless you need to gain body fat, such as an underweight football player. The physique athlete looking to gain muscle while minimizing body fat should focus on whole food nutrition and high-quality protein.

ARE STRENGTH GAINS THE BEST INDICATOR OF MUSCLE GROWTH?

One of the best indicators to gauge progress in the gym is monitoring that your weights and/or reps are increasing. If you are getting stronger each time you go to the gym, don't add additional sets. Although this is a topic of debate among researchers, most studies have found a correlation between

---

180 Alex Ribeiro et al., "Effects of Different Dietary Energy Intake Following Resistance Training on Muscle Mass and Body Fat in Bodybuilders: A Pilot Study," *Journal of Human Kinetics*, February 13, 2019.

strength gains and muscle growth, but this does not always occur.[181] When you exercise, you can get stronger due to improved neurological training (i.e., brain and nervous system) or by building more lean mass. If you are training like a powerlifter and doing singles and doubles, then you can certainly get stronger but more than likely won't build much muscle.

Tracking workout volume is a better gauge of putting on lean muscle mass than just using absolute strength increases.

Most people think that getting stronger means you are adding muscle, but this has not always been the case. For example, two studies found very weak associations between increased muscle mass and strength in a large sample of young, healthy people.[182,183] *This suggests you should not gauge your strength gains as the sole indicator of muscle growth.* Strength gains can occur through neurological improvements and technique rather than increases in muscle size. Improvements in strength can occur because they are getting better at performing the movement rather than increasing muscle size. Strength gains can occur thru training specificity rather than increases in muscle mass. Muscle growth can occur in the absence of changes in strength.[184] It should be mentioned that the more advanced a lifter is, the better the relationship between gains in strength and muscle growth. You are better off tracking lean mass through body composition rather than relying solely on strength gains.

---

181 Carlo Reggiani and Stefano Schiaffino, "Muscle Hypertrophy and Muscle Strength: Dependent or Independent Variables? A Provocative Review," *European Journal of Translational Myology* 30, no. 3 (September 9, 2020): 9311–9311.

182 Juha P. Ahtiainen et al., "Heterogeneity in Resistance Training-Induced Muscle Strength and Mass Responses in Men and Women of Different Ages," *Age* 38, no. 1 (February 2016): 10.

183 Robert M. Erskine, Gareth Fletcher, and Jonathan P. Folland, "The Contribution of Muscle Hypertrophy to Strength Changes Following Resistance Training," *European Journal of Applied Physiology* 114, no. 6 (June 2014): 1239–49.

184 D. G. Sale, J. E. Martin, and D. E. Moroz, "Hypertrophy Without Increased Isometric Strength after Weight Training," *European Journal of Applied Physiology and Occupational Physiology* 64, no. 1 (January 1, 1992): 51–55.

It should be mentioned that beginners rapidly increase muscle strength with no hypertrophy, purely due to neurological improvements. Keep in mind that everyone has a different genetic response to exercise. Some are high responders (i.e., good genetics) and can grow extremely rapidly in response to resistance exercises; contrary to this, there are low-responders (i.e., bad genetics) who make very poor muscle growth, despite doing the same workout.[185] One should only consider adding sets if the muscle you are focusing on is not growing, not feeling an adequate stimulus from the total sets, are experiencing very little fatigue, not getting a good muscle pump, and the set quality is excellent. You should not add sets if you are experiencing fatigue, begin noticing a large reduction in reps from set to set, or have greater than normal post-workout soreness, etc. Slowly add sets to your workout to increase volume rather than making large increases in set volume. If you are training correctly, you should not need more than 3 to 4 sets per exercise, per body part, but it's an individual preference.

ARE YOU A LOW-RESPONDER OR JUST NOT TRAINING CORRECTLY?

There is a term that many people like to use when they don't gain muscle, and that's *"hard gainers."* These people claim that no matter what they do, they can't gain muscle. There is no question that some people, because of poor genetics, don't gain muscle easily. It can be due to several genetic factors:

---

185 Michael D Roberts et al., "Physiological Differences Between Low Versus High Skeletal Muscle Hypertrophic Responders to Resistance Exercise Training: Current Perspectives and Future Research Directions," *Frontiers in Physiology* 9 (July 4, 2018): 834–834.

Genetic factors that you have no control over:

- Myostatin levels (i.e., a gene that reduces muscle growth).

- Lack of satellite cell activation (i.e., satellite cells fuse with muscle fibers to regenerate muscle and is essential for muscle growth).

- Differences in fiber size and type (i.e., people with low type II fibers have difficulty gaining muscle).

- Androgen receptor concentrations in muscle (i.e., low androgen receptor concentration is associated with low muscle growth).

In a study by Dr. Haun, he found that a subject's pre-training muscle fiber size and type determined how much muscle growth they had in response to a six-week resistance exercise protocol. Subjects with the greatest increases in muscle growth had high type II muscle fibers at baseline.[186] Unfortunately, you may not be one of the blessed individuals with an abundance of type II fibers, but there are things you have control over.

Many hard gainers who say they cannot gain muscle often have poor lifestyle choices and training quality that result in subpar muscle growth. Many hard gainers will spend hundreds of dollars on supplements but fail to meet the necessities for gaining muscle. Hard gainers may have certain genetic components that they have no control over, but there are several things that hard gainers *do have control over* that can impact muscle growth:

- Are you eating enough calories to gain muscle?

- Are you consuming sufficient protein to build muscle?

- Are you sleeping enough and resting enough between workouts to gain muscle?

---

186 Cody T. Haun et al., "Pre-Training Skeletal Muscle Fiber Size and Predominant Fiber Type Best Predict Hypertrophic Responses to 6 Weeks of Resistance Training in Previously Trained Young Men," *Frontiers in Physiology* 10 (2019): 297.

- Are you training with too little or too much volume?

- Are you training at the right intensity level (i.e., close to muscular failure)?

- Are you training each body part 2 times per week?

- Are you consistently following a workout plan? (i.e., changing exercises too frequently can reduce program adaptations)

Everyone has a different number of sets to grow. The best example of this was a study in which people who *decreased their sets had better muscle growth*. In this study, subjects were randomly assigned to perform 12, 18, or 24 sets per week for the quads. These were previously trained athletes, so some people increased their sets. In contrast, others decreased their training volume based on their previous sets before entering the study (i.e., some people may have been performing 20 sets per body part before the study and may have been assigned to the 12-set group). Interestingly, the individuals who grew the most increased their number of sets by sets per week, while others gained muscle by reducing their training volume.[187] *It's worth repeating; some subjects gained more muscle by reducing their total training volume.* This points to each person having a unique capacity to recuperate from exercise.

---

187 Daniel Aube et al., "Progressive Resistance Training Volume: Effects on Muscle Thickness, Mass, and Strength Adaptations in Resistance-Trained Individuals," *Journal of Strength and Conditioning Research*, February 13, 2020.

MUSCLEGATE: GERMAN VOLUME TRAINING BUILDS MORE MUSCLE

SAMPLE GERMAN VOLUME TRAINING PROGRAM:

Exercise	Sets	Repitions	Rest
Squats (60% of a 1RM)	10	10	60-90

THE TRUTH EXPOSED: Another classic example of finding the right training volume that works for you is a study investigating German Volume Training (GVT). GVT consists of ten sets of ten repetitions with 1-minute rest periods. When researchers compared subjects who trained with 10 sets of 10 repetitions to 5 sets of 10 repetitions, they found that the low-volume groups (5 sets) had a better increase in muscle growth.[188] There are two issues with GVT, in my opinion. 1.) The research suggests that 5-7 sets are the maximum growth potential for any given exercise. 2.) GVT involves short rest periods (60-90 seconds of rest), which are not conducive for muscle growth (discussed in Chapter 10). Performing 10 sets per body part for an exercise overwhelms the body's ability to recuperate, leading to a sub-optimal muscle growth response. GVT results in what is called junk volume (performing additional sets that are not conducive for muscle growth). I would recommend *RP Scientific Principles of Hypertrophy Training* for an excellent book that discusses training volume.[189] Dr. Mike Israetel has a term he describes as *maximal recoverable volume (MRV)* and *minimal effective volume (MEV)*. MRV is the maximal volume that can be performed *while still recovering*. MEV is the lowest training volume an athlete can do in a particular situation and still measurably improve. Maximum Adaptive Volume (MAV) is the range of volumes you make the

---

188 Theban Amirthalingam et al., "Effects of a Modified German Volume Training Program on Muscular Hypertrophy and Strength," *Journal of Strength and Conditioning Research* 31, no. 11 (November 2017): 3109–19.

189 Dr Mike Israetel M.S, Dr Melissa Davis, Dr James Hoffman, Jared Feather, "Scientific Principles of Hypertrophy Training," 2021.

best gains in muscle growth. Dr. Israetel points out that adding volume comes at the expense of increased recuperation/recovery. MEV is often necessary to give the body a break yet continue to progress.

SAMPLE MEV, MAV, MRV TRAINING CYCLE FROM RP SCIENTIFIC PRINCIPLES OF HYPERTROPHY TRAINING

Week 1: 10-14 sets (Minimal Effective Volume)

Week 2: 12-16 sets (Maximal Adaptive Volume)

Week 3: 14-18 sets (Maximal Adaptive Volume)

Week 4: 16-20 sets (Maximal Recoverable Volume)

Week 5: 6-10 sets (Deload)

Training with high volume is not sustainable for long periods; a break from high-volume training should occur every 4-6 weeks. Notice in the above example, volume increases, followed by a subsequent decline. High-volume workouts cannot occur for prolonged periods. Once you experience fatigue from increased volume, a subsequent reduction in volume should follow. Many lifters don't want to take deloads or training breaks for fear of losing muscle and strength. As you will read later, deloads provide a super-compensation response, in which you will exceed previous training gains. A 2020 study found that a deload week with as little as one set of 6-12 repetitions with an intensity of 70-85% performed 2-3 times per week was sufficient to increase strength.[190] This suggests that bodybuilders and other athletes can take a low volume week to give their bodies added rest and still retain strength gains with as little as one set per muscle group. Once you resume your workout from a deload, start slowly by adding just 1-2 sets per week. Don't make extreme jumps in volume, as this can lead to impaired recuperation. Also, keep in mind that changing exercises will

---

190 Patroklos Androulakis-Korakakis, James P. Fisher, and James Steele, "The Minimum Effective Training Dose Required to Increase 1RM Strength in Resistance-Trained Men: A Systematic Review and Meta-Analysis," *Sports Medicine (Auckland, N.Z.)* 50, no. 4 (April 2020): 751–65.

change the adaptation process and increase muscle soreness. This is best duplicated in the Scarpelli study, in which subjects were assigned to 22 sets per week or a 20% increase in volume each week. The 20% volume increase resulted in greater muscle mass at the end of the study, suggesting a gradual increase in volume is better for muscle growth rather than starting with 22 sets per week.[191]

MUSCLEGATE: DUPLICATE ARNOLD'S ROUTINE TO BUILD MORE MUSCLE

THE TRUTH EXPOSED: It is well documented that Arnold would do anywhere from 20-30 sets for each body part; his legendary marathon routines would last hours. If it worked for Arnold, then it must work for you... right?

SAMPLE ARNOLD SCHWARZENEGGER BACK WORKOUT:

Front wide-grip chin-ups – 6 sets, to failure

T-bar rows – 5 sets, 6-10 reps

Seated pulley rows – 6 sets, 6-10 reps

One-arm dumbbell rows – 5 sets, 6-10 reps

Straight-leg deadlifts – 6 sets, 15 reps

It's no doubt that Arnold had one of the greatest physiques of all time, but this is one person with extremely blessed genetics. Let's look at some of the high set training—20-30 sets—studies per week on muscle gains in regular people. One study had men train three times a week and either did one set per body part or three sets per body part. At the end of the study, the group that did 1 set per week three days a week equaling 9-12 sets per week

---

191 Maíra C. Scarpelli et al., "Muscle Hypertrophy Response Is Affected by Previous Resistance Training Volume in Trained Individuals.," *Journal of Strength and Conditioning Research*, February 27, 2020.

gained more strength and lost more body fat than the group training three sets per week totaling, 27-36 sets per week.[192] In another Arnold-like workout, researchers had subjects gradually increase the number of sets over six weeks. For instance, on week 1, the subjects performed ten sets of squats on week 1, but on week 6, they were performing 32 sets of squats per week! When they tracked muscle growth, muscle growth peaked at roughly ~20 sets per week; after that, the responses plateaued for the group. *The author concluded that ~20 sets per exercise per week is the maximal adaptable training volume for muscle growth.*[193] It should be mentioned that some individuals were still making gains in muscle at 30 sets per week, but the group average plateaued at 20 sets per week. This goes back to the concept mentioned earlier, as there is an upper limit of sets that you can perform while still being able to recuperate, which is unique to each individual. In this case, the subjects after 20 sets were exceeding their maximal recuperation volume. Moderate volume (10 sets per week) is a good place to start is probably the best approach because training volume that is too low or too high can equally impair muscle gains. The average range of sets per week is 10-20 sets per week. Everyone has an individual volume that they can recover from. Don't just copy a superstar's workout plan. For example, I love *The Rock's* motivational videos and his workout drive of getting up at 5 a.m. to train. I saw his workout posted on social media. A typical chest workout for *The Rock* looks like this:

THE ROCK'S WORKOUT PLAN

Incline Dumbbell Bench Press – 4 sets, 12 reps

Alternating Arm Incline Dumbbell Press – 4 sets, 12 reps

---

192 J S Baker et al., "Strength and Body Composition Changes in Recreationally Strength-Trained Individuals: Comparison of One versus Three Sets Resistance-Training Programmes," *BioMed Research International* 2013 (2013): 615901–615901.

193 Cody T. Haun et al., "Effects of Graded Whey Supplementation During Extreme-Volume Resistance Training," *Frontiers in Nutrition* 5 (2018): 84.

Dumbbell Flyes – 4 sets, 15 reps

Dumbbell Bench Press – 4 sets, 12 reps

Alternating Arm Dumbbell Bench Press – 4 sets, 12 reps

Cable Flyes – 3 sets, 25 reps

Dips Until Failure – 4 sets

Total Sets: 28+ Sets per Workout

The research suggests protein synthesis plateaus in the 8-12 sets range.[194] The research also suggests that 6-8 hard sets per bodypart broken up into frequent sessions over the week for a maximum volume of 12-24 sets per bodypart per week is best for muscle hypertrophy.[195] If a person who is not in an advanced training stage and has not adapted his training to this type of volume tries to perform this workout, it would be very difficult to recover from this type of workout. Don't copy superstars' workouts; find a workout that best suits your individual needs.

MORE VOLUME=MORE RECOVERY

Also, keep in mind that high volume, short rest period workouts raise the catabolic hormone cortisol. One study compared a high-volume workout that used 70% of a 1RM (4 sets/10-12 reps/ 1-minute rest periods) to a high-intensity protocol using 90% of a 1RM, which trained with four sets, 3-5 reps, and 3-minute rest periods. At the end of the study, the heavier weight group utilizing longer rest periods resulted in greater gains in strength and lean

---

194 Felipe Damas et al., "Myofibrillar Protein Synthesis and Muscle Hypertrophy Individualized Responses to Systematically Changing Resistance Training Variables in Trained Young Men," *Journal of Applied Physiology (Bethesda, Md.: 1985)* 127, no. 3 (September 1, 2019): 806–15.

195 Daniel Aube et al., "Progressive Resistance Training Volume: Effects on Muscle Thickness, Mass, and Strength Adaptations in Resistance-Trained Individuals.," *Journal of Strength and Conditioning Research*, February 13, 2020.

mass than the high-volume group (5.2% vs. 2.2%). The high-volume, short rest period protocol resulted in greater cortisol responses.[196] This indicates that continuous use of a high-volume/lighter weight/short rest period routine results in a greater physiological stress response than a low-volume, heavy weight protocol with longer rest periods. Another study compared the effects of three different workouts on muscle recovery: 1.) Power (5 sets of 6 at 50% of a 1RM. 2.) Hypertrophy (5 sets-to-failure at 75% of a 1RM, 2-min of rest) and (3) Strength (5 sets-to-failure at 90% of a 1RM, 3-min of rest). The bodybuilding/hypertrophy protocol was found to have the most physiological and perceptual stress compared to the Power and Strength groups. The bodybuilding groups trained with the highest volume reported higher exertion levels and had higher cortisol, lactate, and markers of muscle damage compared to the other groups.[197] This demonstrates that higher volumes are associated with greater physiological stress on the body compared to a heavy weight, low volume protocol. Other studies in animal models have found that when training volume is increased from very low to moderate volume, there is minimal muscle damage. However, when training volume is increased from moderate to high volume, there are large increases in muscle damage.[198] Another study measured muscle recuperation of a powerlifting style, low-volume training routine (8 sets of 3 reps at 90% 1RM with 3 minutes rest between sets) to bodybuilding-style, high-volume training routine with short rest intervals (8 sets of 10 reps at 70% 1RM with 75 seconds rest between sets). The group that trained with a bodybuilding-style workout had suppressed muscle force production (i.e.,

196 Gerald T. Mangine et al., "The Effect of Training Volume and Intensity on Improvements in Muscular Strength and Size in Resistance-Trained Men," *Physiological Reports* 3, no. 8 (August 2015): e12472.

197 André S. Martorelli et al., "The Interplay between Internal and External Load Parameters during Different Strength Training Sessions in Resistance-Trained Men," *European Journal of Sport Science* 21, no. 1 (January 2021): 16–25.

198 M. K. Hesselink et al., "Structural Muscle Damage and Muscle Strength after Incremental Number of Isometric and Forced Lengthening Contractions," *Journal of Muscle Research and Cell Motility* 17, no. 3 (June 1996): 335–41.

a marker of muscle recuperation) for over three days.[199] This means body-building-style workouts result in more muscle soreness, muscle damage, and longer recuperation times. This suggests that volume should not be kept high for prolonged periods of time. Rather, periods of high volume followed by a deload are better for reducing the accumulated stress on the body's nervous and endocrine system.

Contrary to everyone's belief that cortisol is an evil hormone, increases in cortisol are part of the normal muscle growth process. For example, it's been found that there is a positive relationship between post-workout cortisol levels and changes in strength and lean body mass. After 12 weeks of resistance training, researchers found that high post-workout cortisol levels were correlated with gains in lean body mass and changes in type II muscle fiber size.[200] It makes sense that muscle growth correlates with post-exercise cortisol responses since muscle growth involves a stress response. However, chronically high cortisol levels are not conducive for muscle growth and can lead to overtraining. *It is normal for cortisol to increase during exercise and is part of the adaptation process.*

With volume training, as the old saying goes, "The poison is in the dose." One study found in rats that a high volume, high frequency, short rest period training like Arnold trained raised cortisol and decreased muscle size of type I and II fibers.[201]

The problem with prolonged high-volume training is that it can lead to excessive fatigue. Lifting in a fatigued state from excessive training volume results in sub-optimal muscle contractions, elevated stress levels, and

---

199 Sandro Bartolomei et al., "Comparison of the Recovery Response from High-Intensity and High volume Resistance Exercise in Trained Men," *European Journal of Applied Physiology* 117, no. 7 (July 2017): 1287–98.

200 Daniel W. D. West and Stuart M. Phillips, "Associations of Exercise-Induced Hormone Profiles and Gains in Strength and Hypertrophy in a Large Cohort after Weight Training," *European Journal of Applied Physiology* 112, no. 7 (July 2012): 2693–2702.

201 Vinicius Guzzoni et al., "Intense Resistance Training Induces Pronounced Metabolic Stress and Impairs Hypertrophic Response in Hind-Limb Muscles of Rats," *Stress (Amsterdam, Netherlands)* 22, no. 3 (May 2019): 377–86.

depleted energy sources such as glycogen, etc. The key to increasing volume is to pay attention to how you feel. If you add volume and continually feel greater fatigue, it's a good signal to reduce volume. A study found that when comparing a group of men that followed a predetermined workout (example, today train with 85% of a 1RM) or a training session based on monitoring fatigue (example, today I am really tired, I am going to train with 70% of a 1RM) resulted in similar increases in muscle mass, despite the group who monitored fatigue performing less high-intensity workouts.[202] This suggests that monitoring fatigue levels throughout a training cycle optimizes muscle growth.

VOLUME SHOULD BE CYCLED FOR OPTIMAL MUSCLE GROWTH

It should be mentioned that volume should be cycled for optimal muscle growth! Volume is supposed to go through low-volume phases, followed by high-volume stages. A common mistake is to keep volume high throughout a workout cycle; this leads to exhaustion and overtraining. Most experts believe that 10-20 sets are optimal to perform per week for muscle growth. Keep in mind that a considerable amount of overlap occurs for muscle groups like the arms, shoulders, etc. Your arms and deltoids are getting sets added with movements like bench press, bent-over rows, etc. It's better to increase volume for muscle groups like the chest, back, and legs, whereas muscle groups like the arms are getting extra volume from other exercises. A muscle group like the posterior deltoids will need more volume than a muscle group like the anterior deltoids. The anterior deltoid participates in many exercises like the bench press, military press, etc., whereas the posterior deltoid receives less activation. Studies have found

---

202 Rodrigo L. Gomes et al., "Session Rating of Perceived Exertion as an Efficient Tool for Individualized Resistance Training Progression," *The Journal of Strength & Conditioning Research*, October 15, 2021.

that biceps and triceps can increase from doing exercises like bench press and lat pulldowns without any arm workout.

How well you respond to volume depends on your current training program and how much volume you currently perform. Beginners will need to start with low volume, whereas advanced trainers will need more volume. If you are an advanced lifter with several years of experience, start at ten sets per body part. If you are currently performing 10 sets and your muscle growth has plateaued, you can add sets provided your recovery is sufficient. Adding sets above your baseline level can increase muscle growth. To prove my point, researchers took subjects with five years of training experience and had them train legs twice a week. One leg was trained with 22 sets per week, which consisted of leg presses and leg extension. The other leg did the exact exercises but trained with 20% greater volume above their pre-training level. They asked the subjects how many sets they were doing for their normal leg workout. If the subjects were doing ten sets per week (+ 20% increase), the subject would perform 12 sets per week. *Subjects gained more leg growth, on average, in the leg that underwent a 20% volume increase,* even though average volume ended up being similar between conditions.[203] When adding volume, it's best to start with a specific body part you are trying to grow. Adding volume to all body parts can lead to long-term systemic fatigue and an overtraining response.

SAMPLE VOLUME CYCLING WORKOUT FOR A SPECIFIC BODY PART:

1. Start with a low training volume (1-2 sets per body part).

2. Adding 1-2 sets per week.

---

203 Scarpelli, M. C., Nóbrega, S. R., Santanielo, N., Alvarez, I. F., Otoboni, G. B., Ugrinowitsch, C., & Libardi, C. A. (2020). Muscle Hypertrophy Response Is Affected by Previous Resistance Training Volume in Trained Individuals. Journal of strength and conditioning research.

3. Keep doing adding sets each week into your plateau. Your repetition strength falls below baseline, and training exhaustion occurs.

4. Deload and reduce your volume to your beginning set volume of 1-2 sets.

5. Repeat the process.

The purpose of this protocol is to find the maximal volume you can train at and still recover. Once fatigue occurs, you would take a deload and reduce the volume. You would then repeat the process and start adding sets again to determine if you can reach the previous volume you were performing. Once you know the set volume, the maximum stimulus you can train at yet still recover is your *maximal recoverable volume.* The take-home message is to gradually increase set volume rather than start at 20 sets per bodypart a week. Consider volume cycling (changing sets, reps, weight), in which you add sets for a few weeks and then reduce them. Don't freak out by doing less. It's been found that lifters can decrease training volume considerably and not lose muscle.[204] During this time, you provide your body with increased recuperation both psychologically and physiologically.

OLDER LIFTERS NEED MORE RECUPERATION TIME

When addressing the needs of older adults, it's often assumed to do less. Contrary to this notion, older adults need volume to grow just like younger adults. In a 12-week study investigating the effects of failure training in older men, men were divided into three groups:

a. All sets to failure

b. Half the reps taken to failure

---

204 C. Scott Bickel, James M. Cross, and Marcas M. Bamman, "Exercise Dosing to Retain Resistance Training Adaptations in Young and Older Adults," *Medicine and Science in Sports and Exercise* 43, no. 7 (July 2011): 1177–87.

c.   Half the reps to failure but doing more sets.

At the end of the study, despite the older men not training to failure gaining strength, those that performed higher training volume gained more muscle mass. The author concluded that training volume (i.e., groups that trained to failure and groups that performed 50% of reps to failure and more sets) was important for optimizing muscle growth in older adults.[205] Adding volume can be difficult, especially the older athletes. It's been documented that older people have greater muscle damage after exercise and slower muscle recovery than younger adults.[206] Your training volume should be reduced as you get older to accommodate adequate recovery between workouts.

In the words of the great eight-time Mr. Olympia Lee Haney, "Stimulate Don't Annihilate Muscles." The key to adding sets is not to have excess muscle damage. As mentioned previously, everyone has a different genetic capacity to recover. There are people who experience exaggerated muscle damage, inflammation, and slower recovery in response to exercise based on their genetics.[207,208] Too little volume will not be effective, and too much volume will be counterproductive to muscle growth. The process of building muscle involves more protein synthesis than protein breakdown. If you are constantly breaking down muscle tissue, you will not increase muscle growth.

---

205 Larissa Xavier Neves da Silva et al., "Repetitions to Failure versus Not to Failure during Concurrent Training in Healthy Elderly Men: A Randomized Clinical Trial," *Experimental Gerontology* 108 (July 15, 2018): 18–27.

206 P. M. Clarkson and M. E. Dedrick, "Exercise-Induced Muscle Damage, Repair, and Adaptation in Old and Young Subjects," *Journal of Gerontology* 43, no. 4 (July 1988): M91-96.

207 Monica J. Hubal et al., "CCL2 and CCR2 Polymorphisms Are Associated with Markers of Exercise-Induced Skeletal Muscle Damage," *Journal of Applied Physiology (Bethesda, Md.: 1985)* 108, no. 6 (June 2010): 1651–58.

208 Anna Thalacker-Mercer et al., "Cluster Analysis Reveals Differential Transcript Profiles Associated with Resistance Training-Induced Human Skeletal Muscle Hypertrophy," *Physiological Genomics* 45, no. 12 (June 17, 2013): 499–507.

THE FOLLOWING FACTORS DETERMINE TRAINING VOLUME:

- Training Age: Older adults recover slower and therefore need fewer sets

- Training Volume is different by muscle groups. Some muscle groups like the arms and anterior deltoids are used in many exercises and require less volume than those like the chest.

- Beginners should start with a low training volume.

- Advanced lifters will need a higher training volume.

- Longer rest periods (~3 minutes or greater) will allow for greater training volume.

- A larger training volume will require longer recuperation. It's best to split workouts up over the week to achieve a greater training volume.

- Higher workout intensity will cause lower training volume.

- Your current training volume will determine how many additional sets you can add while recuperating

CHAPTER SUMMARY:

- Volume (i.e., sets) has a strong relationship with hypertrophy.

- Hypertrophy can occur with a wide range of set volumes. This is highly dependent on your genetics, ability to recuperate, and current training status.

- Sets must be taken close to failure to result in optimal muscle growth.

- The more sets performed to failure, the greater the muscle damage.

- Studies have found that repeatedly going to failure in each set can lead to less muscle growth.

- Muscle damage is separate from muscle growth.

- Excess muscle damage will impair the muscle growth process.

- Strength increases should not be the sole indicator of muscle growth.

- The number of sets you can perform is dependent on your recovery. Increasing sets will work up to a certain point; then, no further increase in muscle mass will occur.

- The research suggests that between 10-20 sets per body part seems optimal.

- Multiple sets increase muscle protein synthesis and anabolic signaling pathways in muscle compared to single sets.

- Volume has an inverted U-shaped relationship in which sets can increase muscle growth up to a point. Thereafter, adding further sets won't increase muscle growth.

- High volume training can raise cortisol levels and result in excess muscle damage.

- Older adults need more recuperation time.

- The number of sets is a better driver of muscle growth than the weight used when exercise intensity is sufficiently high.

- Muscle growth can occur from a range of weights lifted from 30% to 85% of a 1RM.

- Well-trained athletes need more volume for muscle growth.

- Volume should be cycled with periods of a deload.

- Each person has a unique recovery capacity to resistance exercise.

CHAPTER 6:
REPETITION SPEED & NUMBER OF REPETITIONS FOR OPTIMAL MUSCLE GROWTH

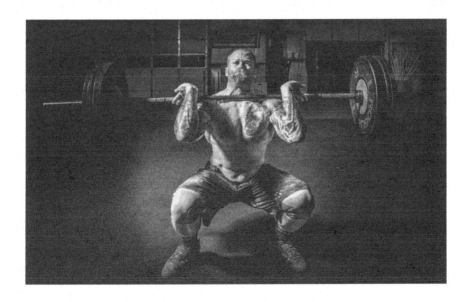

There is intense debate about the optimal repetition speed to perform to maximize muscle growth. Most books and magazines recommend lifting the weight with a slow and controlled lifting speed to maximize tension on the muscle. This led to the rise of SUPERSLOW training, which emphasizes an exaggerated slow lifting speed to maximize tension. Unfortunately, it's not effective for maximizing muscle growth.

MUSCLEGATE: REPETITIONS MUST BE PERFORMED SLOWLY TO GAIN MUSCLE

THE TRUTH EXPOSED: If you read any fitness book, it will state that repetitions should be performed in a slow, controlled manner for optimal muscle growth. In the early '90s, there was training called *"SUPER SLOW,"* which advocated taking 10 seconds to lift the weight and lowering the weight in 10 seconds. The theory is that slower lifting results in greater *time under tension (TUT)*.

TUT is defined as the amount of time a muscle is contracting by timing the duration of the sets and reps. TUT is highly controversial among researchers because it's hard to quantify. If you raise and lower the weight slower, more tension is placed on the muscle. Sounds reasonable, but unfortunately, the claims don't hold up to the science. Remember that aerobic exercise involves low tension for long periods, but very little to no muscle growth occurs of Type II fibers. If you are looking to grow muscle, you need to think about the amount of time under tension that can stimulate high threshold type II muscle fibers that are the most capable of muscle growth. The muscle-building stimulus does not strictly rely on the length of each set, but the amount of weight lifted and how close to failure each set is performed. In the previous chapter, it was discussed that a certain effort of intensity of effort threshold that must be met to increase muscle growth. SuperSlow incorporates a much lighter weight than is typically used for increasing muscle growth. As a result of using an extremely light weight, it reduces the total tension placed on the muscle, resulting in sub-optimal muscle growth. Remember from the previous chapter that intensities <30% resulted in subpar muscle growth when taken to failure. If time under tension were the determining factor for muscle growth, one would expect longer TUT to result in superior muscle growth, but research does not support this. For example, one study compared a bodybuilding protocol using (3 sets of 10 repetitions), whose TUT was 30-40 seconds to a powerlifting protocol (7 sets of 3 reps) with a TUT of 9-12 seconds resulted in similar muscle growth.[209] If TUT were the predominant muscle growth stimulus, one would expect the bodybuilding protocol to gain more muscle, but this did not occur. One of the predominant factors for muscle growth is muscular tension. Using a SuperSlow with light weight will not place enough tension on the muscle to optimally stimulate muscle growth! Remember, total volume is a function of sets x reps x weight. If the weight is reduced to train with SuperSlow, then the total volume is being reduced. You will likely generate too much fatigue before optimal muscle tension is placed on the muscle for growth stimulus. This should bring awareness to the so-called 100-rep squat protocol to grow your legs. Light weight protocols to failure can increase muscle growth, but it's much more painful to perform and results in high fatigue, whereas heavier weight can be performed short of failure and still increase muscle growth.

HOW LONG SHOULD REPETITIONS LAST FOR MUSCLE GROWTH?

Some studies have found that lifting weight slowly can contribute to muscle growth. Still, most research suggests that muscle growth can occur at a wide range of repetition durations that can range from .8 to 8 seconds.[210] Training at volitionally very slow repetition durations (>10's seconds per repetition) is inferior for muscle hypertrophy. A 2021 study compared muscle growth in response to fast repetitions (1-second concentric, 0-second isometric, 1-second eccentric) versus slow (1-second concentric, 0-second isometric, 3-second eccentric) repetitions in the leg muscles. The total volume was equal between the groups. *At the end of the study, there was no difference in muscle size between the two groups.* The fast group had a

---

209 Talisson Santos Chaves, Thaís Marina Pires de Campos Biazon, Lucas Marcelino Eder dos Santos, et al., ~Effects of Resistance Training with Controlled versus Self-Selected Repetition Duration on Muscle Mass and Strength in Untrained Men," ed. Gerald Mangine, *PeerJ* 8 (March 6, 2020): e8697.

210 Brad J. Schoenfeld, Dan I. Ogborn, and James W. Krieger, "Effect of Repetition Duration during Resistance Training on Muscle Hypertrophy: A Systematic Review and Meta-Analysis," *Sports Medicine (Auckland, N.Z.)* 45, no. 4 (April 2015): 577–85.

greater increase in muscles in certain leg parts.[211] This suggests that when total training volume is similar, it does not matter how fast or slow the repetitions are; it's an individual preference. This sum collection of studies suggests you should not worry about the repetition tempo, as muscle growth can occur in a wide range of lifting tempos. Just lift the weight you feel is a comfortable pace for you. Repetition speed can be anywhere from .8 to 8 seconds to achieve muscle growth. Repetition speeds lasting longer than 10 seconds have been found to be inferior for muscle growth.

THERE IS A WIDE RANGE OF REPETITION SPEEDS TO STIMULATE MUSCLE GROWTH

It does not seem to matter if you slow down the lifting tempo if the total volume between the groups is similar. A 2020 study reported that when one group lifted with a 2-second concentric and a 2-second eccentric phase compared to a group that lifted at a much quicker repetition speed resulted in similar increases in muscle growth.[212] The author concluded, "***When the total work volume is identical, lifting at a self-selected repetition speed, regardless of the tempo, resulted in similar increases in strength and muscle.***" Another 2021 review of the literature concluded that slow lifting movements did not enhance muscle growth. The author concluded that, despite lowering the weight slowly, which increases time under tension, the lower amount of weight utilized often led to a lower total training volume. Based on the research, lifting tempo has a minor effect on muscle growth. Still, it seems more favorable for muscle growth to use a combination of

---

211 Jeremy Pearson et al., "Does Varying Repetition Tempo in a Single-Joint Lower Body Exercise Augment Muscle Size and Strength in Resistance-Trained Men?," *The Journal of Strength & Conditioning Research*, 9000.

212 Chaves, T. S., Pires de Campos Biazon, T. M., Marcelino Eder Dos Santos, L., & Libardi, C. A. (2020). Effects of resistance training with controlled versus self-selected repetition duration on muscle mass and strength in untrained men. PeerJ, 8, e8697.

slower eccentric movements paired with faster concentric movements.[213] You should perform each exercise with a weight that feels comfortable to you if the exercise duration is no longer than ~8 seconds. Keep in mind that when using *SuperSlow*, the tension on the muscle is low, and the high threshold muscle fibers that experience the greatest muscle growth will not be activated at the beginning of the set; they will only be activated toward the end of the set. In contrast, a moderate to heavy weight will recruit those high threshold muscle fibers *faster at the beginning of the set.*

SUMMARY: Lifting the weight slower does not seem to significantly affect muscle growth when volume is similar between groups. Lifting the weight slowly often reduces the total workout volume (i.e., sets x weight x reps) by using a lighter weight than usual. Slower movement tempos decrease the external load; however, if the movements are taken to muscular failure, they can create an adequate stimulus to induce muscle growth. However, it's still more time-efficient to use a moderately heavy weight because it activates more fast-twitch fibers sooner.

MUSCLEGATE: TO GAIN MORE MUSCLE, REPETITIONS MUST BE PERFORMED WITH 8–10 REPS

THE TRUTH EXPOSED: There has been a complete reexamination of the so-called "hypertrophy zone." It was typically thought that repetitions less than 5 increase strength (80-100% of a 1RM), repetitions between 8-12 stimulate muscle growth (60-80% of a 1RM), and repetitions greater than 15 optimize endurance (60% of a 1RM). The new research suggests that *muscle growth can occur at a wide range of repetitions; there is no magic number, there is no "hypertrophy zone."* Lopez et al. analyzed over

---

213 Michal Wilk, Adam Zajac, and James J. Tufano, "The Influence of Movement Tempo During Resistance Training on Muscular Strength and Hypertrophy Responses: A Review," *Sports Medicine (Auckland, N.Z.)* 51, no. 8 (August 2021): 1629–50.

28 studies investigating muscle growth in response to various rep ranges. Only studies in which sets were performed to volitional failure were included. Studies comprised of a wide variety of rep ranges, including high – (>15 repetitions maximum (RM), moderate – (9-15 RM), and low (≤8 RM) resistance training. The author concluded that in untrained – and recreationally trained individuals, muscle hypertrophy or muscle growth was *load or weight-independent*. Strength gains only occurred by using a heavier weight.[214] He also found that those with more years of training (2-7 years) needed more sets and reps to gain muscle. A 2021 meta-analysis of 23 studies with 563 participants found that heavier weights increased maximal strength. In contrast, a wide spectrum of loads or weight (30-90%) can be used for muscle hypertrophy. The author also stated that heavier weights can cause excessive wear and tear on the joints and ligaments; therefore, alternating between light, moderate, and heavy loads is a good strategy for muscle hypertrophy.[215] More resistance training sessions are necessary for those with a longer training experience, providing greater increases in muscle size due to a principle of diminishing return. Untrained athletes can gain muscle with as little as 3-5 sets per week, but muscle growth will eventually plateau if you continue to use this set range. The more trained you are, the more volume you will need to grow.

A recent study by Kubo et al. examined the effects on muscle size and strength in 42 men assigned to four groups: One group did seven sets of 4 reps each session, one group did 4 sets of 8 reps, and one group did 3 sets of 12 reps. *Irrespective of the rep range used, muscle size was similar between all the groups.* It should also be mentioned that the 4 and 8 rep groups had greater increases in strength than the 12-rep group. The author

---

214 Pedro Lopez et al., "Resistance Training Load Effects on Muscle Hypertrophy and Strength Gain: Systematic Review and Network Meta-Analysis," *Medicine and Science in Sports and Exercise* 53, no. 6 (June 1, 2021): 1206–16.

215 Marcio Lacio et al., "Effects of Resistance Training Performed with Different Loads in Untrained and Trained Male Adult Individuals on Maximal Strength and Muscle Hypertrophy: A Systematic Review," *International Journal of Environmental Research and Public Health* 18, no. 21 (January 2021): 11237.

suggested that if you are looking for the best of both worlds of increasing size and strength, it's probably best to use rep ranges between 6-8 repetitions.[216] Training with moderate (8-12 reps) and high reps (25-35 reps) to failure results in similar increases in muscle growth.[217]

It should also be noted that anything less than four reps is not conducive to muscle growth; more than likely, the volume will be low to stimulate muscle growth. Remember, there is an inverse relationship between volume and intensity. Heavier weights will reduce training volume (i.e., reps x sets). It was found that when comparing a bodybuilding type protocol of 8-12 reps to a strength protocol of 2-4 reps, the bodybuilding protocol built more muscle. In contrast, the low rep group built more strength.[218] It's been suspected that training with heavy weights, low-rep sets (< 6 reps) do not place the muscle under tension long enough to stimulate muscle growth adequately. When subjects were required to perform one rep maximal strength training for 21 days, it did not increase muscle growth, suggesting that a single repetition of high tension is insufficient to stimulate muscle growth.[219] Also, keep in mind that heavier weight training will stress joints and ligaments. One study compared lifters training with a 3-repetition maximum (powerlifting protocol) compared to a 10-repetition maximum (bodybuilding protocol) for eight weeks. Both groups had equal gains in muscle mass when the volume was equated, but it should be mentioned that the 3RM powerlifting group experienced more joint pain and had a

---

216 Keitaro Kubo, Toshihiro Ikebukuro, and Hideaki Yata, "Effects of 4, 8, and 12 Repetition Maximum Resistance Training Protocols on Muscle Volume and Strength," *The Journal of Strength & Conditioning Research* 35, no. 4 (2021).

217 Brad J. Schoenfeld et al., "Effects of Low – vs. High-Load Resistance Training on Muscle Strength and Hypertrophy in Well-Trained Men," *Journal of Strength and Conditioning Research* 29, no. 10 (October 2015): 2954–63.

218 Brad J. Schoenfeld et al., "Differential Effects of Heavy Versus Moderate Loads on Measures of Strength and Hypertrophy in Resistance-Trained Men," *Journal of Sports Science & Medicine* 15, no. 4 (December 2016): 715–22.

219 Scott J. Dankel et al., "Muscle Adaptations Following 21 Consecutive Days of Strength Test Familiarization Compared with Traditional Training," *Muscle & Nerve* 56, no. 2 (August 2017): 307–14.

higher dropout rate due to injury.[220] This suggests that using heavier weight will increase the risk of injury and should be used sparingly, as muscle growth is your primary goal. Another study of interest compared a body-building protocol consisting of 4 sets of 8-12 reps to failure and a group that performed maximal strength testing with 5 maximal attempts every day. The group that performed the hypertrophy workout had the advantage of increasing muscle size in multiple muscle regions to max strength testing every day.[221] The sum collection of the studies suggests that training with powerlifting type protocols with low reps does not place the muscle under tension for enough time to create optimal increases in muscle. Training with blocks of heavier weight for longer periods results in added stress to the joints. Still, similar muscle growth can occur by using a lighter weight with more reps, provided the reps are taken close to failure. What if your goal is to develop more power? Athletes need peak explosive power to maximize performance. What does the research suggest that the optimal repetitions speed is for gaining peak power?

LIFT FASTER FOR EXPLOSIVE POWER

If you are attempting to get *stronger*, the research suggests that you lift and lower the weight slightly faster than normal resistance exercise. By using high-velocity momentum during lifts, athletes can improve their power production by using explosive movements with high tension. Lifting a heavy load at high speed facilitates the recruitment of high threshold motor units. Davies et al. performed a meta-analysis of 15 studies. They found that studies in which subjects lifted quickly (1-second concentric and 1-second eccentric) gained greater strength compared to moderate to

220 Brad J. Schoenfeld et al., "Effects of Different Volume-Equated Resistance Training Loading Strategies on Muscular Adaptations in Well-Trained Men," *Journal of Strength and Conditioning Research* 28, no. 10 (October 2014): 2909–18.

221 Kevin T. Mattocks et al., "Practicing the Test Produces Strength Equivalent to Higher Volume Training," *Medicine and Science in Sports and Exercise* 49, no. 9 (September 2017): 1945–54.

slow repetition speed.[222] If you have ever watched Olympic lifter's train, it's amazing to see how fast they perform the clean and jerk and snatch. They do all their exercises explosively! One of the most exciting technologies to be utilized by strength coaches for improving performance is *velocity-based training*. It allows a user to see how fast the barbell was lifted in real-time. They can try to lift the barbell more quickly and gauge their performance.

GETTING MORE EXPLOSIVE POWER AND MINIMIZING FATIGUE

Velocity-based training has emerged as a practical alternative to resistance training intensity (% of an RM). Velocity-based training provides velocity ranges to base the workout around rather than maximally load the bar with weights. Velocity-based training improves power because a maximal effort is required for all reps of all sets. Therefore, much of the strength gains result from increased access to high-threshold muscle fibers. It has been recognized that providing feedback to athletes (e.g., lift the bar more explosively) as they train can enhance velocity and power outputs by up to 10%.[223]

Velocity-based training is also a great way to measure fatigue during a set. The closer the set is to failure, the greater the velocity loss. Applying velocity loss thresholds can limit the amount of fatigue induced in a training cycle and control training volume, depending on the training goal. It has been found that there is a correlation between velocity loss, lactate (linear relationship), and ammonia concentration, meaning the greater the velocity loss, the greater the fatigue and metabolic response.[224] In a recent

222 Timothy B. Davies et al., "Effect of Movement Velocity During Resistance Training on Dynamic Muscular Strength: A Systematic Review and Meta-Analysis." *Sports Medicine (Auckland, N.Z.)* 47, no. 8 (August 2017): 1603–17.

223 Jonathon Weakley et al., "Velocity-Based Training: From Theory to Application," *Strength and Conditioning Journal* 43 (April 1, 2021): 31–49.

224 Luis Sánchez-Medina and Juan José González-Badillo, ~Velocity Loss as an Indicator of Neuromuscular Fatigue during Resistance Training," *Medicine and Science in Sports and Exercise* 43, no. 9 (September 2011): 1725–34.

meta-analysis of velocity loss, it was concluded that applying velocity loss of 10-20% can reduce fatigue and help induce neuromuscular adaptations. Velocity zones can elicit positive changes in body composition and improve performance parameters.[225] Velocity feedback during training motivates athletes to achieve better results and keeps them accountable for their performance. They can see in real-time exactly how much velocity was generated with each lift. A recent study compared velocity-based training to traditional resistance training found that the velocity-based training group had improved maximal strength and jump height, despite using a lower total workload.[226] It should be mentioned that a meta-analysis of velocity-based training of six different studies found that both % based training (i.e., % 1RM) and velocity-based training were equally effective for increasing strength, jump performance, linear spring, and change of direction.[227]

STOPPING SHORT OF FAILURE RESULTS IN GREATER STRENGTH GAINS

There is evidence that stopping short of failure results in greater strength gains. Researchers had participants perform bench press (80-100% of a 1RM) with a fast velocity but stopped each set when the velocity dropped > 20%. The group did not perform more sets when the velocity of the first repetition of a new set fell > 20% (i.e., did not train to failure). Another group continued bench press training to complete muscular failure. Despite the non-failure group performing 62% fewer repetitions, the

225 Michał Włodarczyk et al., "Effects of Velocity-Based Training on Strength and Power in Elite Athletes—A Systematic Review," *International Journal of Environmental Research and Public Health* 18, no. 10 (January 2021): 5257.

226 Harry F. Dorrell, Mark F. Smith, and Thomas I. Gee, "Comparison of Velocity-Based and Traditional Percentage-Based Loading Methods on Maximal Strength and Power Adaptations," *Journal of Strength and Conditioning Research* 34, no. 1 (January 2020): 46–53.

227 Kai-Fang Liao et al., "Effects of Velocity Based Training vs. Traditional 1RM Percentage-Based Training on Improving Strength, Jump, Linear Sprint and Change of Direction Speed Performance: A Systematic Review with Meta-Analysis," *PloS One* 16, no. 11 (2021): e0259790.

maximal velocity group improved bench press maximal strength by 10.2%, whereas the group training to failure resulted in a meager < 1%. This suggests that measuring the individual performance speed for each set can be useful for increasing strength gains.[228] Another study compared changes in lean mass and strength with velocity losses of 20 or 40% in males after eight weeks using the squat. A 40% velocity loss implies performing repetitions to, or very close to, muscle failure in most exercise sets. In contrast, a 20% velocity loss corresponds to performing approximately half the maximum number of repetitions per set, which means the 20% velocity loss group trained further away from failure than the 40% velocity loss group. The 20% velocity loss group had similar squat strength gains to the 40% velocity loss group, and greater improvements in jumping performance (9.5% vs. 3.5%), despite the 20% velocity loss group performing 40% fewer repetitions. However, in terms of muscle growth, the 40% velocity loss group resulted in more fatigue and metabolic stress, resulting in greater hypertrophy of the quads. Interestingly, the 20% velocity loss group still increased quadriceps growth, despite performing ~58% of the training volume performed by 40% velocity loss.[229] It can be suggested that the greater tension, metabolic stress, and greater volume contributed to the greater increases in muscle growth in the 40% velocity group. It also suggests that training to failure is not conducive to strength gains in advanced lifters and, managing fatigue contributes to increased peak power. A 2021 study found that when subjects trained with six exercises with a strength workout (i.e., 5 sets of 5 reps to failure) had greater strength loss than training with a group training with a power workout (i.e., 5 sets of 50% of a 5RM), despite both groups using the same total workload. Recovery for the strength training group was not complete 48 hours after exercise, whereas moderate-load recovery

228 J. Padulo et al., "Effect of Different Pushing Speeds on Bench Press," *International Journal of Sports Medicine* 33, no. 5 (May 2012): 376–80.

229 F. Pareja-Blanco et al., "Effects of Velocity Loss during Resistance Training on Athletic Performance, Strength Gains and Muscle Adaptations," *Scandinavian Journal of Medicine & Science in Sports* 27, no. 7 (July 2017): 724–35.

required less than 48 hours.[230] This suggests that training to failure will result in prolonged recovery time. Training to failure even when the volume is similar to non-failure training, each set led to reduced bench press and squat strength and resulted in recovery for up to three days, whereas stopping short of failure can result in recovery within 48 hours.[231] Training to failure results in diminished training frequency and volume during a training week due to impaired recovery between workouts.

SUMMARY: If you want to gain power, lift weights explosively to teach your nervous system to fire faster. If you look at Olympic lifters, you will never find them lifting the weight slowly. Olympic lifting focuses on lifting the weight as explosively as possible while maintaining a strict form. Using velocity-based training or other visual feedback is a great way to improve power by lifting with the greatest maximal effort for each rep while minimizing fatigue. Training closer to failure is better for gains in lean mass. However, better strength gains are achieved when stopping well before failure.

CHAPTER SUMMARY:

- Lifting tempo is highly variable for muscle growth that can occur at a wide range of repetition durations ranging from .8 to 8 seconds.

- Changing lifting tempo is a good idea. Much of the research suggests that a faster lifting tempo favors muscle growth.

---

230 Christian Helland et al., "A Strength-Oriented Exercise Session Required More Recovery Time than a Power-Oriented Exercise Session with Equal Work," *PeerJ* 8 (September 30, 2020): e10044.

231 Ricardo Morán-Navarro et al., ~Time Course of Recovery Following Resistance Training Leading or Not to Failure,~ *European Journal of Applied Physiology* 117, no. 12 (December 2017): 2387–99.

CHAPTER 7:
TRAINING TO FAILURE

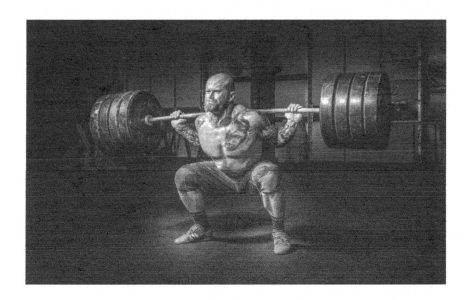

TRAINING TO FAILURE: THE PROS AND CONS

Based on what you have read so far, many of you probably realize that there is a relationship between fatigue, volume, and muscle growth. If you read carefully, *most of the research to date advocates you train close to failure or near failure but not to complete muscular failure.* If you have read any fitness magazine or bodybuilding book in the past decade, it usually advocated training to complete muscular failure each set for muscle growth. Some bodybuilding gurus recommended even training past the point of failure by having your workout partner assist you in doing additional reps once fatigued. A good way of judging how close you are approaching failure is to gauge how fast the concentric portion of the lift slows each additional repetition. Despite being advocated for promoting muscle growth, new research suggests that sometimes, it may be best to stop a few reps short of failure.

MUSCLEGATE: TRAIN TO COMPLETE MUSCULAR FAILURE FOR MORE MUSCLE GROWTH

THE TRUTH EXPOSED: Training to failure is an enormous debate among researchers and trainers alike. It's confusing because earlier in the chapter, you have read that most studies suggest that training close to or near failure is essential for muscle growth. Training to failure takes an enormous toll on the muscular and nervous system. Studies have found that training to complete muscular failure increases muscle fatigue and decreases performance in the subsequent sets.[232,233] This means that the subsequent intensity of the workout will be further reduced in each set because of fatigue. Training to failure results in cellular depletion of substrates. Subjects training to failure marked a decrease in power output during the last 5 repetitions of each set. This was accompanied by an 80% fall in phosphocreatine and a 21% drop in ATP levels. Subjects that did half the reps and stopped before failure had a 15% drop in phosphocreatine levels and no depletion of ATP levels and maintained power output throughout the entire training protocol.[234] On a cellular level, training to failure elicits a greater cellular toll on the body.

232 Sanmy R. Nóbrega et al., ~Effect of Resistance Training to Muscle Failure vs. Volitional Interruption at High – and Low-Intensities on Muscle Mass and Strength," *Journal of Strength and Conditioning Research* 32, no. 1 (January 2018): 162–69.

233 Natalia Santanielo et al., "Effect of Resistance Training to Muscle Failure vs Non-Failure on Strength, Hypertrophy and Muscle Architecture in Trained Individuals," *Biology of Sport* 37, no. 4 (December 2020): 333–41.

234 Esteban M. Gorostiaga et al., "Energy Metabolism during Repeated Sets of Leg Press Exercise Leading to Failure or Not," *PLOS ONE* 7, no. 7 (July 13, 2012): e40621.

Training to failure each set is also going to extend recuperation time. Researchers tested strength and workout capacity following eight sets of bench press to failure and subjects repeated the workout at 24-, 48-, 72-, and 96-hours following training. Subjects' maximal strength was decreased for 72 hours; furthermore, their ability to perform their baseline work capacity was still decreased for 96 hours.[235] It has been demonstrated that training to failure caused sustained fatigue and performance drops the following day in the bench press (-7.2%) and half-squat (-11.1%), whereas there were no performance drops when training two reps shy of failure the previous day.[236] This suggests that going to failure on each set will prolong your ability to retrain that muscle again. What if you train with most of your sets away from failure, but take the last set to failure? Researchers compared two bench press programs using 80% of a 1-RM completing five sets. One group trained to complete failure each set, whereas the other group trained short of failure (i.e., 3 RIR) but did the last set until complete muscular failure (0 RIR). A progressive decline in repetitions, work completed, and barbell velocity was seen across sets taken to complete muscular failure. In contrast, when subjects stopped approximately within 3 repetitions of failure for a majority of their sets, overall barbell velocity was greater, completed repetitions and work were more consistent across sets and perceived effort of exercise stress was less.[237] This suggests that if you feel you must train to failure, minimize it to one set, as the effects are lesser than taking every set to failure.

235 Diogo V. Ferreira et al., "Dissociated Time Course between Peak Torque and Total Work Recovery Following Bench Press Training in Resistance Trained Men," *Physiology & Behavior* 179 (October 1, 2017): 143–47.

236 Domingo Ramos-Campo et al., "Effects of Resistance Training Intensity on the Sleep Quality and Strength Recovery in Trained Men: A Randomized Cross-over Study," *Biology of Sport* 38 (August 1, 2020).

237 Gerald T. Mangine et al., "Effect of the Repetitions-In-Reserve Resistance Training Strategy on Bench Press Performance, Perceived Effort, and Recovery in Trained Men," *The Journal of Strength & Conditioning Research* 36, no. 1 (January 2022): 1–9.

PROS AND CONS OF

FAILURE

VS

NON-FAILURE TRAINING

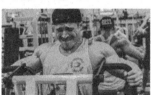

		FAILURE	NON-FAILURE
	RECOVERY	Greater Recovery	Less Recovery
	MULTIJOINT EXERCISE	Greater Injury Potential	Less Injury Potential
	SINGLE JOINT EXRCISE	Less Injury	-
	FATIGUE	Greater Fatigue	Less Fatigue
	MUSCLE GROWTH	Less Muscle Growth for Advanced	Greater Muscle Growth for Advanced
	WEIGHT	~ 30% of a 1RM Should Be Taken to Failure	60-80% of a 1RM Not Necessary
	PROTEIN SYNTHESIS	Increased with light weight training (~30% of a 1RM)	Decreased with light weight training (~30% of a 1RM)
	FREQUENCY	Training Each Body Part Once per Week	Training Each Body Part 2 X Per week
	LAST WEEK OF TRAINING BEFORE A DELOAD	👍	👍

Several studies have found that training to complete muscular failure was superior to traditional training for muscle growth. However, earlier research studies used untrained or somewhat trained subjects, and the total training volume was higher in the training to failure groups (i.e., more reps) which led to greater muscle mass. In athletes who combine resistance training with specific sports training, it seems rational to not train to failure each set, considering stopping short of failure results in similar or even greater muscle strength and power gains compared with resistance training to failure[238]. Recent studies have found that for *trained subjects,* training just shy or close to muscular failure is better for muscle growth than training to failure each set.[239] The most recent 2021 meta-analysis of training to failure vs. not training to failure found that *there does not appear to be an overall benefit of training to failure for strength or muscle growth.*[240]

BEGINNERS, NOT ADVANCED LIFTERS, SHOULD TRAIN TO FAILURE

It is recommended that beginners train to failure; *however, intermediate and advanced lifters are recommended to train shy of failure for most of their training sessions.* It is recommended that in the last week of training of a mesocycle, all sessions be taken to complete muscular failure. It is worth repeating, the only time you should train to complete failure is the last week before a deload in which the volume and intensity of exercise will be reduced. As mentioned previously, training to complete muscular failure

---

238 Alexandra F. Vieira et al., "Effects of Resistance Training Performed to Failure or Not to Failure on Muscle Strength, Hypertrophy, and Power Output: A Systematic Review With Meta-Analysis," *Journal of Strength and Conditioning Research* 35, no. 4 (April 1, 2021): 1165–75.

239 Tim Davies et al., "Effect of Training Leading to Repetition Failure on Muscular Strength: A Systematic Review and Meta-Analysis," *Sports Medicine (Auckland, N.Z.)* 46, no. 4 (April 2016): 487–502.

240 Alexandra F. Vieira et al., "Effects of Resistance Training Performed to Failure or Not to Failure on Muscle Strength, Hypertrophy, and Power Output: A Systematic Review With Meta-Analysis," *Journal of Strength and Conditioning Research* 35, no. 4 (April 1, 2021): 1165–75.

results in impaired recovery; therefore, a deload the week after the final week of a training cycle, where you are exerting maximal effort makes sense. It's also recommended that smaller isolation exercises like biceps curls and calf raises can be taken closer to failure than compound movements such as the squat and deadlift.

All the collective new research suggests that minimizing going to complete failure for each set is better for gaining muscle. It's commonly recommended that each set be stopped with one or two reps before reaching complete muscular failure. Muscle activation (i.e., EMG activity) of the quads was similar between 70, 80, and 90% of back squat 1RM with slightly greater values at maximal effort (100% of 1RM). This suggests that near-maximal muscle activation can occur in the 0-4 RIR range (i.e., training close to failure) when using multi-joint movements.[241] It can be theorized to manage fatigue, as volume increases over the weeks, start with lower RIR (i.e., 4-5 RIR) and gradually move closer to a 0-1 RIR as the weeks progress. Slowly increase workout stress instead of starting a workout cycle at 0-1 RIR (i.e., near maximal effort) and risk overtraining with excessive exercise intensity early in the mesocycle.

MUSCLEGATE: TRAIN TO FAILURE WITH HEAVY WEIGHT FOR MORE MUSCLE GROWTH

THE TRUTH EXPOSED: *You can train anywhere from 60–80% of a 1-RM and not train to failure and gain as much muscle as those that train to failure.*[242] This goes back to the research that suggests that you don't have to leave the gym completely wiped out to grow. A study found that when two groups trained with the same volume, the group that used a

---

241 van den Tillaar, R., Andersen, V., & Saeterbakken, A. H. (2019). Comparison of muscle activation and kinematics during free-weight back squats with different loads. *PloS one*, *14*(5), e0217044.

242 Sanmy R. Nóbrega and Cleiton A. Libardi, "Is Resistance Training to Muscular Failure Necessary?," *Frontiers in Physiology* 7 (January 29, 2016): 10.

combination of heavy and light weights (i.e., relative intensities based on sets and repetitions) gained more muscle than those who trained with repetition maximums and went to failure each workout.[243] The author suggested that heavy weight training to failure resulted in excess fatigue, reduced ability to adapt, and reduced recovery. The excess fatigue led to a lesser muscle growth response compared to the relative intensity group not training to failure.

It may be confusing since, in the earlier chapters, it was mentioned there was research suggesting that training closer to failure resulted in more muscle growth. The big difference in studies comparing muscle growth to training to failure vs. non-training failure is heavily flawed because the training to failure group uses more volume (i.e., reps). One study compared 2 groups of individuals in which one group trained to failure and the other did not but used a similar total workload. The non-failure group did an additional set to ensure the total workload was similar between the groups. *When the volume is equated at the end of the study, the non-training group gained equal muscle strength, hypertrophy, and muscular endurance.*[244] This suggests that the earlier studies that had subjects train to failure had more muscle growth because they performed more volume. Still, the research that equated exercise protocols found that training shy of failure can result in similar muscle growth.

During the big compound lifts like squats, deadlifts, bench press, and overhead press, you want to train a few reps shy of failure most of the time. However, you can train to failure for single-joint exercises such as bicep curls, calf raises, triceps extensions, etc. This is due to greater central and peripheral fatigue using compound movements as opposed to

---

243 Kevin M. Carroll et al., "Skeletal Muscle Fiber Adaptations Following Resistance Training Using Repetition Maximums or Relative Intensity," *Sports* 7, no. 7 (July 2019): 169.

244 Saulo Martorelli et al., "Strength Training with Repetitions to Failure Does Not Provide Additional Strength and Muscle Hypertrophy Gains in Young Women," *European Journal of Translational Myology* 27, no. 2 (June 24, 2017): 6339.

isolation exercises. Typical training sessions should be taken close (i.e., 2 reps away from complete muscular failure) or when you notice that there is a measurable loss in the speed of your repetitions. Just how far away you can stop short of failure is debatable, but most experts recommend 1 to 2 reps shy of muscular failure for compound exercises. Remember that the minimum time needed to recuperate muscles when performing ten sets to failure would be 72 hours.[245] Overall, some muscles tolerate higher workout volumes than others while training with the same frequency.[246] For example, after maximal sprints, the hamstrings can take longer to recover than the quadriceps after intense exercise. Quadriceps strength returned to baseline strength levels at 48 hours, whereas hamstring strength was still not recovered.[247]

TRAINING TO FAILURE RESULTS IN A DETERIORATION IN FORM

Another common issue with training to failure is a loss of training form. Olympic lifters always use reps of < 5 because excess fatigue results in a deterioration of movement form. Remember that when you train to complete muscular failure, it's not uncommon to shift body positions inadvertently (i.e., exercise form) to help you achieve the repetition. This change in body position will shift the attention from the desired working muscle to other muscles. For example, it's not uncommon to shift the barbell to a lower position on the back during the squat to lift the weight when highly fatigued. The primary purpose of squats is to train the quadriceps. By

245 Karine Naves De Oliveira Goulart et al., "Time-Course of Changes in Performance, Biomechanical, Physiological and Perceptual Responses Following Resistance Training Sessions," *European Journal of Sport Science* 21, no. 7 (July 2021): 935–43.

246 Trevor C. Chen et al., "Damage and the Repeated Bout Effect of Arm, Leg, and Trunk Muscles Induced by Eccentric Resistance Exercises," *Scandinavian Journal of Medicine & Science in Sports* 29, no. 5 (May 2019): 725–35.

247 Philipp Baumert et al., "Neuromuscular Fatigue and Recovery after Strenuous Exercise Depends on Skeletal Muscle Size and Stem Cell Characteristics," *Scientific Reports* 11, no. 1 (April 8, 2021): 7733.

shifting the weight to the lower back, you activate more lower back, glutes, and hamstrings, resulting in less quadriceps activation.[248] It's much easier to maintain proper form with single-joint exercises to fatigue, such as the preacher curl and triceps extension, than multi-joint exercises such as bench press, deadlifts, and squats. If you have ever watched a person squat to complete muscular failure, it's not uncommon to see exercise form rapidly deteriorate the last few reps. It may be wise to use single-joint exercises to failure to maintain exercise form instead of risking injury with improper form due to high fatigue with complex multi-joint movements requiring high coordination. Exercise fatigue can alter technique, which determines how much tension is placed on the muscle. Never sacrifice exercise form and risk injury at the expense of repetitions. The factors that are going to influence the amount of fatigue sustained during a workout are: the number of reps (i.e., high reps result in greater fatigue), the rest period between sets (i.e., shorter rest periods result in more fatigue), and if the reps are taken to complete muscular failure.

WHEN YOU SHOULD TRAIN TO FAILURE

There are times when you should train to failure, and that's if you are using light weights. One study compared training to failure with light (30% of a 1RM) and heavy weight (90% of a 1RM) but also had a group that trained light (30%) and stopped short of failure. The group that stopped short of failure had inferior protein synthesis rates than the light and heavy weight group training to failure.[249] Light weight taken to failure (i.e., > 30% of a 1RM) results in similar muscle growth to heavy weight taken to failure,

---

248 Tae-Sik Lee, Min-Young Song, and Yu-Jeong Kwon, "Activation of Back and Lower Limb Muscles during Squat Exercises with Different Trunk Flexion," *Journal of Physical Therapy Science* 28, no. 12 (December 2016): 3407–10.

249 Burd, N. A., West, D. W., Staples, A. W., Atherton, P. J., Baker, J. M., Moore, D. R., Holwerda, A. M., Parise, G., Rennie, M. J., Baker, S. K., & Phillips, S. M. (2010). Low-load high volume resistance exercise stimulates muscle protein synthesis more than high-load low volume resistance exercise in young men. PloS one, 5(8), e12033.

but sub-par muscle growth occurs when light weights are used and not taken to failure. It has also been found that bench pressing with a light weight (40 percent 1RM) to failure and doing bodyweight push-ups to failure (twice a week 3 sets to failure) resulted in similar muscle growth between the two exercises.[250] When most people think of high rep training, they make the mistake of thinking that because it is light weight, they can recuperate faster. Light weight training takes longer to recuperate from than heavy weight training. When researchers compared a heavy weight program (80% of a 1RM) to a light-weight training program (30% of a 1RM), fatigue persisted longer after the light-weight training program. The author concluded you get more bang for your buck with heavier weight training because heavier weight usage results in greater muscle activation during training with fewer repetitions.[251] This suggests that if you plan a high-rep, metabolic stress training day, plan for more recuperation time after your workout.

Another instance where it's beneficial to train to failure is training each muscle group once a week. Training to failure will prolong muscle recuperation time, but if you are training each muscle group once per week, this will not be an issue. Training once a week is not optimal for muscle growth, but if you insist on training once a week, take each set to failure.

When to Train to Failure:

- **Training a body part once a week**

- **Training with a very light weight (i.e., 30% of a 1RM)**

- **At the end of a training cycle, before a deload**

---

250 Naoki Kikuchi and Koichi Nakazato, "Low-Load Bench Press and Push-up Induce Similar Muscle Hypertrophy and Strength Gain," *Journal of Exercise Science and Fitness* 15, no. 1 (June 2017): 37–42.

251 Cody T. Haun et al., "Molecular, Neuromuscular, and Recovery Responses to Light versus Heavy Resistance Exercise in Young Men," *Physiological Reports* 5, no. 18 (September 2017): e13457.

- Isolation exercises with low risk of technical execution
- A beginner just starting to exercise

MUSCLEGATE: INCREASES IN GH AND TESTOSTERONE BOOSTS MUSCLE GROWTH

THE TRUTH EXPOSED: You have already learned that it's unnecessary to train to failure, and there is no difference in muscle growth between those going to failure and those who do not. Studies suggest that when monitored over a period of weeks, *not training to failure* is better for anabolic hormones. Izquierdo and colleagues found that training to failure resulted in suppressed levels of muscle-building hormones (i.e., reduced IGF-1 levels). In contrast, the non-training failure group had lower cortisol levels and higher testosterone levels.[252] Cortisol can block anabolic signaling events in the muscle and interfere with the binding of testosterone to receptors in the muscle.[253] Therefore, it is essential to keep cortisol in balance and allow for recovery for optimal training and subsequent adaptations.

Training to failure increases growth hormone, testosterone, and cortisol (i.e., catabolic hormone) acutely or in the short term, *but training to failure reduces testosterone in the long term.* The impact of whether the acute increases in GH and testosterone affect muscle growth is debatable. The combined effects of resistance exercise and exercise-induced anabolic hormones may lead to an upregulation of anabolic signaling pathways, which likely augments net protein synthesis and hypertrophy.[254] However,

---

252 Mikel Izquierdo et al., "Differential Effects of Strength Training Leading to Failure versus Not to Failure on Hormonal Responses, Strength, and Muscle Power Gains," *Journal of Applied Physiology* 100, no. 5 (2006): 1647–56.

253 Barry A. Spiering et al., "Effects of Elevated Circulating Hormones on Resistance Exercise-Induced Akt Signaling," *Medicine and Science in Sports and Exercise* 40, no. 6 (June 2008): 1039–48.

254 Nima Gharahdaghi et al., "Links Between Testosterone, Oestrogen, and the Growth Hormone/Insulin-Like Growth Factor Axis and Resistance Exercise Muscle Adaptations," *Frontiers in Physiology* 11 (2021): 1814.

a vast majority of the studies suggest that acute increases in anabolic hormones have no impact on muscle growth. Professor Stuart Phillips has led the charge on debunking the role of acute anabolic hormones and muscle growth. In a 2016 study, subjects trained with either a heavy weight, low repetitions (~75%-90% of a 1RM), or high repetitions (~30–50% of a 1RM). Despite an acute increase in anabolic hormones, there was no correlation between acute anabolic hormones and muscle growth; both groups increased muscle mass similarly.[255] One exciting finding from this study was that local androgen receptor concentration was correlated with increased muscle mass, suggesting that rather than systemic hormones (i.e., testosterone, GH), androgen receptor concentration is more important for muscle growth.

The current research suggests that acute anabolic hormones play a lesser role in muscle growth than previously thought. Subjects were trained with either arm curls (low anabolic hormone exposure) or arm curls plus leg press and leg extension/leg curl at ~90% of 10 RM (high anabolic hormone levels). It has been well documented that large multi-joint exercises like the leg press produce greater anabolic hormones than smaller joint exercises like the bicep curls. If acute anabolic hormones led to muscle growth, the arms training with leg training that resulted in greater anabolic hormone exposure should have resulted in greater muscle growth. Despite arms plus legs workouts producing large increases in GH, testosterone, and IGF-1 levels, they found no differences in the arm size exercised under low or high anabolic hormone conditions after 15 weeks of training.[256] Based on the sum collection of all the studies, the acute anabolic hormone rise

255 Robert W. Morton et al., "Neither Load nor Systemic Hormones Determine Resistance Training-Mediated Hypertrophy or Strength Gains in Resistance-Trained Young Men," *Journal of Applied Physiology* 121, no. 1 (July 1, 2016): 129–38.

256 Daniel W. D. West et al., "Elevations in Ostensibly Anabolic Hormones with Resistance Exercise Enhance Neither Training-Induced Muscle Hypertrophy nor Strength of the Elbow Flexors," *Journal of Applied Physiology* 108, no. 1 (January 2010): 60–67.

from exercise has a minor effect on muscle growth.[257] One study found that after 12 weeks of resistance training, the resistance exercise changes in testosterone had no direct correlation with muscle fiber growth.[258] Keep in mind that women can gain substantial increases in muscle size in response to a resistance exercise program, despite having lower testosterone levels than men.[259] If the acute increases in GH were a contributing factor to the muscle growth process, one would expect that training in the morning in which the body's naturally occurring GH levels are higher would result in more muscle growth. The study's sum collection does not show that training in the morning is more effective than in the afternoon for muscle growth, despite having higher GH in the morning.[260] More than likely, you don't need to worry about the acute anabolic effects of testosterone and GH in response to exercise and muscle growth. Tension on the muscle is more important than the acute anabolic hormone response.

MUSCLEGATE: FORCED REPS CAUSE MORE MUSCLE GROWTH

THE TRUTH EXPOSED: It's very common to see lifters use a spotter to assist them with the last few reps of a set. Based on the above finding that reps taken to failure do not result in more muscle growth than sets that are stopped several reps short of failure, I have little faith that forced

---

257 E. Todd Schroeder et al., "Are Acute Post–Resistance Exercise Increases in Testosterone, Growth Hormone, and IGF-1 Necessary to Stimulate Skeletal Muscle Anabolism and Hypertrophy?," *Medicine & Science in Sports & Exercise* 45, no. 11 (November 2013): 2044–51.

258 G. E. McCall et al., "Acute and Chronic Hormonal Responses to Resistance Training Designed to Promote Muscle Hypertrophy," *Canadian Journal of Applied Physiology = Revue Canadienne de Physiologie Appliquee* 24, no. 1 (February 1999): 96–107.

259 Monica J. Hubal et al., "Variability in Muscle Size and Strength Gain after Unilateral Resistance Training," *Medicine and Science in Sports and Exercise* 37, no. 6 (June 2005): 964–72.

260 Jozo Grgic et al., "The Effects of Time of Day-Specific Resistance Training on Adaptations in Skeletal Muscle Hypertrophy and Muscle Strength: A Systematic Review and Meta-Analysis," *Chronobiology International* 36, no. 4 (April 2019): 449–60.

reps will stimulate more muscle growth. There is no study to date that has examined forced reps' responses to traditional exercise for muscle hypertrophy. Still, I would assume that it would be similar to the training to failure vs. non-failure training, which favors non-failure training. A 2003 study found that forced reps resulted in greater GH and increased cortisol responses than a traditional resistance exercise protocol. This means that there was greater workout stress associated with forced reps. Recovery time after the workout was prolonged in the forced rep group for three days post-exercise.[261] Forced reps result in greater recuperation time between workouts. Forced reps also cause greater peripheral and central fatigue. Furthermore, forced reps have not been found to increase strength compared to traditional resistance exercises.[262]

---

261 J. P. Ahtiainen et al., "Acute Hormonal and Neuromuscular Responses and Recovery to Forced vs. Maximum Repetitions Multiple Resistance Exercises," *International Journal of Sports Medicine* 24, no. 6 (August 2003): 410–18.

262 Eric J. Drinkwater et al., "Increased Number of Forced Repetitions Does Not Enhance Strength Development with Resistance Training," *Journal of Strength and Conditioning Research* 21, no. 3 (August 2007): 841–47.

CHAPTER SUMMARY:

- Trained subjects training just shy or close to muscular failure is better for muscle growth than training to failure each set.

- Training to complete muscular failure increases muscle fatigue and recuperation time between workouts.

- Training to failure with heavy weight does not seem beneficial in the long term.

- You can train anywhere from 60–80% of a 1-RM and not train to failure and gain as much muscle as those that train to failure.

- If you are using an extremely light weight (<30% of a 1RM), train to failure.

- Light weight training (30% of a 1-RM) stopping short of failure had inferior protein synthesis rates compared to light and heavy weight group training to failure.

- Acute anabolic hormones (GH and testosterone) do not impact muscle growth.

- Forced reps result in increased cortisol and more muscle damage.

- <1-minute rest periods reduce muscle protein synthesis and muscle growth.

CHAPTER 8:

FATIGUE &
RECOVERY MANAGEMENT

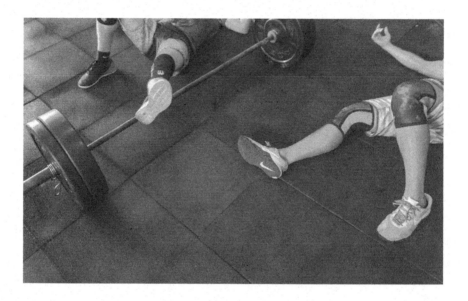

Many lifters know what recovery means, but they don't truly grasp the severity of the relationship between fatigue and muscle growth. Recovery can be defined as a restoration of physiological systems to baseline before further overloading a muscle again. ***Muscle growth occurs during recovery!*** If you are not recovering between workouts, don't expect to make significant gains in muscle growth or strength. One study found that constantly stimulating a muscle without sufficient rest increased oxidative stress (i.e., cellular stress) and *suppressed increases in protein synthesis*

rates after exercise.[263] Remember, building muscle is a function of increasing protein synthesis while minimizing protein breakdown. If you are constantly breaking down muscle, you are not growing! Your body will eventually become overly fatigued by continuous exercise if you don't take a break or deload. For example, one study found that biceps growth was *lower* with 27 weekly sets compared to 18 sets. This suggests that after 18 sets, the fatigue response was too great, and no further training could stimulate muscle growth.[264] As mentioned previously, this is an example of junk volume in which further sets than required are no longer are conducive to muscle growth. The key is to find the right balance of stimulus to fatigue ratio before repeating the process. Everyone has a different genetic ability to recover from exercise; therefore, each person's workout program should be unique to that person. Also, your ability to recuperate is highly dependent on your diet. A recent review of 17 studies found that physical performance can be *maintained* when consuming a ketogenic diet compared with carbohydrate diets. However, *the current evidence does not support an ergogenic effect of consuming a ketogenic diet.*[265] If you are not gaining muscle over the course of your training, the workout stress is too high, and you are not taking sufficient rest to recover between workouts. Conversely, your workout stress may be too low, and you are not stimulating the muscle enough to enhance muscle growth, or you are not consuming enough calories, not sleeping enough, etc.

Many people are quick to neglect the optimal amount of sleep they need for muscle growth. A 2017 study of over 10,125 university students found that those who slept less than 6 hours had poorer strength than

---

263 Junya Takegaki et al., "Repeated Bouts of Resistance Exercise with Short Recovery Periods Activates MTOR Signaling, but Not Protein Synthesis, in Mouse Skeletal Muscle," *Physiological Reports* 5, no. 22 (November 2017): e13515.

264 Samuel R. Heaselgrave et al., "Dose-Response Relationship of Weekly Resistance— Training Volume and Frequency on Muscular Adaptations in Trained Men," *International Journal of Sports Physiology and Performance* 14, no. 3 (March 1, 2019): 360–68.

265 Murphy, N. E., Carrigan, C. T., & Margolis, L. M. (2021). High-Fat Ketogenic Diets and Physical Performance: A Systematic Review. Advances in nutrition (Bethesda, Md.), 12(1), 223–233.

those who slept 7-8 hours.[266] Furthermore, a single night of sleep loss can increase cortisol by 24%, reduce testosterone by 24%, and reduce protein synthesis by 18%.[267] Researchers found that when subjects slept 1 hour less a night for five days resulted in a substantial loss of muscle compared to a group that was allowed a normal sleep pattern.[268]

TYPES OF FATIGUE

Most people don't know this, but different types of fatigue can occur during exercise: central and peripheral fatigue. Resistance exercise can cause both central and peripheral fatigue.[269] For an excellent review on the role of muscle growth and fatigue, one should read Chris Beardsley's book: *Hypertrophy: Muscle fiber growth caused by mechanical tension.*[270]

Central fatigue or systemic fatigue is most associated with aerobic exercise; it is associated with the brain and spinal cord. If your brain is fatigued, you will have problems performing a maximal contraction. Ever watch a long-distance runner in the last few miles? You may notice that he has coordination problems; this is an example of central fatigue. Your brain is causing muscles to contract; if your brain and central nervous system are tired, you won't generate a maximal force. Psychological fatigue from the daily stressors of life can also affect performance. Studies have found that when subjects had to perform complex math equations before squats, there

---

266 Yanbo Chen et al., "Relationship between Sleep and Muscle Strength among Chinese University Students: A Cross-Sectional Study," *Journal of Musculoskeletal & Neuronal Interactions* 17, no. 4 (December 2017): 327–33.

267 Séverine Lamon et al., "The Effect of Acute Sleep Deprivation on Skeletal Muscle Protein Synthesis and the Hormonal Environment," *Physiological Reports* 9, no. 1 (January 5, 2021): e14660.

268 Xuewen Wang et al., "Influence of Sleep Restriction on Weight Loss Outcomes Associated with Caloric Restriction," *Sleep* 41, no. 5 (May 1, 2018).

269 Adam Zając et al., "Central and Peripheral Fatigue During Resistance Exercise – A Critical Review," *Journal of Human Kinetics* 49 (December 22, 2015): 159–69.

270 Beardsley, C. Hypertrophy: Muscle fiber growth caused by mechanical tension. 2019

was a decrease in the training volume they could perform.[271] This was also found when people used social media before exercise; this also resulted in reduced exercise performance compared to a control group.[272] This is just an example of how mental fatigue can impair weightlifting performance.

Peripheral fatigue or local fatigue during exercise results in metabolic accumulation in muscles such as lactate, calcium, etc. Metabolic stress from high-intensity exercise and muscle damage causes central fatigue and peripheral fatigue. Also, training to complete muscular failure results in more peripheral fatigue and may cause more muscle damage.[273] Single-leg exercises elicit greater peripheral fatigue than double leg exercises. For example, single-leg extensions resulted in greater peripheral fatigue than double-leg extensions.[274] Most people think heavy weight, high-intensity exercise causes more central fatigue, but low-intensity, high volume exercise causes greater central fatigue.[275] In this study, researchers compared training with 20% of a 1RM and 80% of a 1RM to failure in both men and women. Central fatigue was greater for both men and women with the 20% contraction to failure than the 80%. If you have ever done a squat for >30 reps, you know it is extremely taxing on the body. It's also been found that compound movements can cause greater central fatigue than single-joint

271 "Mental Fatigue Reduces Training Volume in Resistance Exercise: A Cross-Over and Randomized Study – Victor Sabino de Queiros, Matheus Dantas, Leonardo de Sousa Fortes, Luiz Felipe Da Silva, Gilson Mendes Da Silva, Paulo Moreira Silva Dantas, Breno Guilherme de Araújo Tinôco Cabral, 2021,~ accessed October 8, 2021.

272 Leonardo Fortes et al., "Effects of Social Media on Smartphone Use before and during Velocity-Based Resistance Exercise on Cognitive Interference Control and Physiological Measures in Trained Adults," *Applied Neuropsychology: Adult*, December 29, 2020.

273 Jorge M. González-Hernández et al., ~Resistance Training to Failure vs. Not to Failure: Acute and Delayed Markers of Mechanical, Neuromuscular, and Biochemical Fatigue," *Journal of Strength and Conditioning Research* 35, no. 4 (April 1, 2021): 886–93.

274 Matthew J. Rossman et al., "The Role of Active Muscle Mass in Determining the Magnitude of Peripheral Fatigue during Dynamic Exercise," *American Journal of Physiology. Regulatory, Integrative and Comparative Physiology* 306, no. 12 (June 15, 2014): R934-940.

275 Tejin Yoon et al., "Mechanisms of Fatigue Differ after Low – and High-Force Fatiguing Contractions in Men and Women," *Muscle & Nerve* 36, no. 4 (October 2007): 515–24.

exercises, so performing compound movements *first* can ensure that you maximize your workouts.[276] Fatigue must be managed during exercise to increase workout volume. It's well documented that high volume training to failure results in prolonged recuperation time between workouts and exacerbates muscle damage. One of the primary symptoms of overtraining/overreaching is reduced strength and fatigue. This likely occurs in part due to central nervous system fatigue-reducing muscle force output.

---

276 Matthew J. Rossman et al., "The Role of Active Muscle Mass in Determining the Magnitude of Peripheral Fatigue during Dynamic Exercise," *American Journal of Physiology. Regulatory, Integrative and Comparative Physiology* 306, no. 12 (June 15, 2014): R934-940.

TYPES OF FATIGUE DURING EXERCISE

Central Fatigue

Brain and Spinal Cord

Central fatigue is defined as a reduction in the ability to voluntarily activate a muscle during a maximal effort.

- Inflammation
- CNS Fatigue
- Muscle Damage

EXERCISE FACTORS:

- High Repetitions
- Short Rest Periods
- Large Muscle Groups

Peripheral Fatigue

Muscle

Peripheral fatigue refers to a reduction in the ability of the muscles to produce force, regardless of the signal from the central nervous system.

- Metabolite Accumulation (Lactate, Hydrogen Ions)
- Metabolite Depletion (ATP, Creatine Phosphate)

EXERCISE FACTORS:

- Single Joint Exercises

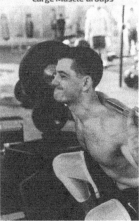
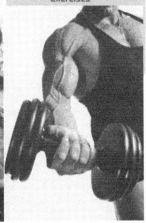

TRAINING TO FAILURE CAUSES MORE FATIGUE AND LONGER RECOVERY

Think of building muscle, like building a brick wall. You go to the gym (i.e., sledgehammer) and cause damage to that wall. The builder then repairs (i.e., protein synthesis) and adds new bricks (i.e., muscle growth). Using that sledgehammer more (i.e., training to failure) causes more damage, and it takes longer for that builder to repair the wall. Direct damage to the muscle after exercise causes inflammation and prolongs muscle recovery time.[277] It has also been found that training to failure can contribute to overuse injuries. An individual's muscle fiber types (i.e., fast twitch or slow twitch) can also determine whether they recuperate faster or slower. Athletes with more fast-twitch fibers are more likely to overtrain. One study found that when athletes were exposed to an overtraining period, it caused some to overtrain while others did not. The athletes that experienced overtraining had more fast-twitch explosive fibers. Those athletes with more fast-twitch fibers will result in more fatigue than those with slow-twitch fibers. Athletes with more fast-twitch fibers demonstrated fatigue for a maximal 90-second exercise bout for 5 hours after exercise, whereas athletes with the slow-twitch fibers had recovered 20 minutes after exercise.[278] Athletes with more fast-twitch fibers will experience more fatigue than those with slow-twitch fibers. This suggests that your genetic makeup of fibers can determine whether you can handle a high-volume program or not. Remember, not all athletes respond to every workout the same; no cookie-cutter weight training program works for everyone.

As mentioned, not all muscle groups recover at the same rate. Slow-twitch fibers will recuperate at a faster rate than fast-twitch fibers. Therefore, you can train the calves, which comprise a high proportion of

277 Arthur J. Cheng, Baptiste Jude, and Johanna T. Lanner, "Intramuscular Mechanisms of Overtraining," *Redox Biology* 35 (August 2020): 101480.

278 Eline Lievens et al., "Muscle Fiber Typology Substantially Influences Time to Recover from High-Intensity Exercise," *Journal of Applied Physiology* 128, no. 3 (March 1, 2020): 648–59.

type I fibers, more frequently than a muscle group like the hamstrings, which consist primarily of type II fibers and take longer to recover. The calf soleus muscle is about 80% type I muscle fiber (i.e., soleus Type I fibers range from 64 to 100%). In contrast, the gastrocnemius and vastus lateralis muscles only contain 57% slow-twitch fibers (range 34–82%).[279] A well-planned training cycle will have a high stimulus-to-fatigue ratio, placing high tension on the muscle without overly fatiguing the nervous system. An example of a high stimulus to fatigue ratio technique would be using the mind-muscle connection, actively squeezing the muscle with each rep, and stopping with 1-2 RIR. Lots of muscle stimulation while minimizing fatigue. In contrast, going to failure each set results in a worse stimulus to fatigue ratio because you are causing excess fatigue with no added stimulation. Another example of a worsening stimulus to fatigue ratio would be high rep squats with light weight. This generates extreme fatigue when squats performed with a heavier weight can achieve the same results with less fatigue stopping short of failure.

MASKING FATIGUE

Many lifters mask their fatigue by taking large amounts of caffeine and other pre-workout stimulants. It's well documented that pre-workout stimulants can increase performance by enhancing mood and vigor, increasing repetitions to fatigue, and increasing total workout volume.[280] The big issue is that excessive pre-workouts can mask symptoms of overtraining and chronic fatigue. In my experience, I have seen lifters needing 2–3 scoops of a pre-workout before workouts to mask fatigue. Caffeine can reduce

---

279 Philip D. Gollnick et al., "Human Soleus Muscle: A Comparison of Fiber Composition and Enzyme Activities with Other Leg Muscles," *Pflügers Archiv* 348, no. 3 (September 1, 1974): 247–55.

280 Patrick S. Harty et al., "Multi-Ingredient Pre-Workout Supplements, Safety Implications, and Performance Outcomes: A Brief Review," *Journal of the International Society of Sports Nutrition* 15, no. 1 (August 8, 2018): 41.

pain perception during exercise.[281] It has also been found that caffeine can decrease muscle soreness by 22%.[282] It could be suggested that with increasing levels of muscle damage and fatigue, lifters are self-medicating with caffeine to continue exercising when they should reduce their training load. The other issue is that many lifters will take a pre-workout after work when they go to the gym, disrupting sleep. A study found that taking 400 mg of caffeine six hours before bedtime disrupted sleep quality.[283] Those who train at night after work should consider a stim-free workout or a pre-workout with a low amount of caffeine. Think again if you don't think sleep will impact your muscle growth gains! A recent study that took lifters and taught them sleep optimization techniques resulted in greater increases in muscle mass than the group that performed the same resistance exercise program.[284] I have no issues with pre-workouts with increasing performance, but don't abuse pre-workout to mask symptoms of fatigue, and it's probably best to cycle pre-workouts. For example, only use pre-workouts the last few weeks in which maximal effort is required. You don't need a pre-workout when starting a new training cycle and going light.

MAXIMIZING RECOVERY WITH NUTRITION

Muscle growth involves a stimulus, fatigue, resistance, and finally, exhaustion. Building muscle is highly individualized; some people recover faster and slower than others. Recovery depends on a wide range of variables such

281 Jozo Grgic et al., "The Influence of Caffeine Supplementation on Resistance Exercise: A Review," *Sports Medicine* 49, no. 1 (January 2019): 17–30.

282 Hou-Yu Chen et al., "Effects of Caffeine and Sex on Muscle Performance and Delayed-Onset Muscle Soreness after Exercise-Induced Muscle Damage: A Double-Blind Randomized Trial," *Journal of Applied Physiology* 127, no. 3 (September 1, 2019): 798–805.

283 Christopher Drake et al., "Caffeine Effects on Sleep Taken 0, 3, or 6 Hours before Going to Bed," *Journal of Clinical Sleep Medicine : JCSM : Official Publication of the American Academy of Sleep Medicine* 9, no. 11 (November 15, 2013): 1195–1200.

284 Pål Jåbekk et al., ~A Randomized Controlled Pilot Trial of Sleep Health Education on Body Composition Changes Following 10 Weeks~ Resistance Exercise,~ *The Journal of Sports Medicine and Physical Fitness* 60, no. 5 (May 2020): 743–48.

as genetics, nutrition, sleep, etc. Athletes quickly try out the latest training recovery modalities, such as ice baths, foam rolling, and infrared therapy, but forget about the basics. With the ongoing low and keto carb craze phenomenon, many athletes fail to realize that maximizing glycogen stores with carbohydrate-rich diets is essential for recuperation.[285] Adequate carbohydrates will also reduce muscle tissue breakdown. Low carbohydrates are worse for increasing lean muscle mass than a high-carbohydrate diet.[286] Cutting carbs not only reduces your ability to recover properly but reduces your ability to train at higher intensities and volume the following day. In a study of CrossFit athletes, athletes who had performance decline associated with overtraining had three times lower carbohydrates than healthy CrossFit athletes.[287] In a recent meta-analysis of overtraining syndrome, 18 out of 21 studies observed reductions in performance because of inadequate energy or carbohydrate intake rather than excessive training load.[288]

Depending on how hard you are training, most lifters will need 1–3 grams of carbohydrate per pound of body weight. Protein intake should be close to 1–1.5 grams per pound of body weight. This also depends on what kind of daily activity you have. If you have a physically demanding job, you will need more calories than someone who sits at a computer all day. It's best to consume a majority of your carbohydrates directly after exercise to maximize glycogen replenishment. Consuming proteins with carbohydrates enhances glycogen synthesis following exercise, a finding that has

---

285 John L. Ivy, "Regulation of Muscle Glycogen Repletion, Muscle Protein Synthesis and Repair Following Exercise," *Journal of Sports Science & Medicine* 3, no. 3 (September 1, 2004): 131–38.

286 Salvador Vargas et al., "Efficacy of Ketogenic Diet on Body Composition during Resistance Training in Trained Men: A Randomized Controlled Trial," *Journal of the International Society of Sports Nutrition* 15, no. 1 (July 9, 2018): 31.

287 Flavio A. Cadegiani, Claudio E. Kater, and Matheus Gazola, "Clinical and Biochemical Characteristics of High-Intensity Functional Training (HIFT) and Overtraining Syndrome: Findings from the EROS Study (The EROS-HIFT)," *Journal of Sports Sciences* 37, no. 11 (June 3, 2019): 1296–1307.

288 Trent Stellingwerff et al., "Overtraining Syndrome (OTS) and Relative Energy Deficiency in Sport (RED-S): Shared Pathways, Symptoms and Complexities," *Sports Medicine (Auckland, N.Z.)* 51, no. 11 (November 2021): 2251–80.

implications for speeding recovery.[289] Also, it's best to keep fat intake low directly after training because consuming fats with carbohydrates slows glycogen replacement. It has been reported that high-fat feeding post-exercise can impair muscle protein synthesis and anabolic signaling pathways (i.e., p70S6K), potentially causing maladaptive training adaptation responses if performed long term.[290] A highly detailed scientific paper on offseason dieting for bodybuilders suggested that bodybuilders looking to gain muscle while minimizing excessive fat gain consume:

Calories: A slightly hyper-energetic diet (~10–20% above maintenance calories) with the aim of gaining ~0.25–0.5% of body weight per week.

Protein: Protein intake is recommended to be .7–1 gram per pound of body weight per day with a focus on sufficient protein at each meal (minimum of 20 grams) and an even distribution throughout the day (3–6 meals).

Fat: Fats should be consumed at moderate levels, neither too low nor high (.2–.7 grams per pound of body weight per day), to prevent an unfavorable change in free testosterone ratios and to prevent reductions in testosterone levels.

Carbohydrates: After calories have been devoted to protein and fat, the remaining calories should come from carbohydrates while ensuring sufficient amounts are consumed (≥1.3–2.2 grams per pound per day).[291]

---

289 John L. Ivy, "Regulation of Muscle Glycogen Repletion, Muscle Protein Synthesis and Repair Following Exercise," *Journal of Sports Science & Medicine* 3, no. 3 (September 1, 2004): 131–38.

290 Kelly M. Hammond et al., "Postexercise High-Fat Feeding Suppresses P70S6K1 Activity in Human Skeletal Muscle," *Medicine and Science in Sports and Exercise* 48, no. 11 (November 2016): 2108–17.

291 Juma Iraki et al., "Nutrition Recommendations for Bodybuilders in the Off-Season: A Narrative Review," *Sports* 7, no. 7 (June 26, 2019): 154.

SINGLE VS. MULTI-JOINT EXERCISE RECOVERY

Muscle growth has been found to occur earlier with single-joint exercises due to the movements being easier to perform and less neural adaptations. Complex movements that require more neural stimulation have a delayed hypertrophy response.[292] A few papers have examined recovery times for single vs. multi-joint exercises. Remember, there is a large variability in how people recuperate from exercise. Some people recuperate faster or slower than others. One study examined a full-body workout that consisted of either 3 or 7 sets of a 10-repetition maximum. All the sets were taken to complete muscular failure. Many of the subjects who did 3 sets were fully recovered by 48 hours. However, there was large variability among the subjects. For example, after 48 hours of recovery, only 4 of the subjects were fully recovered enough to duplicate their initial performance, while 8 of the subjects recovered fully after 72 hours of rest. One subject had still not recovered after 72 hours! When the researchers increased the sets to 7, subjects needed 96 hours of recuperation before their strength returned to baseline.[293] This was only seven sets per exercise! You can imagine what happens to recovery when you boost that to 20 sets.

A similar study did a whole-body workout consisting of one set of eight reps with 85% of a 10-RM and then one set to failure a 10-RM. 80% of the subject's strength returned to baseline by 48 hours; however, multi-joint exercises such as the squat and deadlift took longer to recover. It should be mentioned that of the ten exercises measured (i.e., barbell bench press, deadlift, military dumbbell press, leg press, knee extension, machine chest fly, triceps extension, dumbbell side raises, hip adduction, hip abduction,

---

292 P. D. Chilibeck et al., "A Comparison of Strength and Muscle Mass Increases during Resistance Training in Young Women," *European Journal of Applied Physiology and Occupational Physiology* 77, no. 1–2 (1998): 170–75.

293 John R. McLester et al., "A Series of Studies--a Practical Protocol for Testing Muscular Endurance Recovery," *Journal of Strength and Conditioning Research* 17, no. 2 (May 2003): 259–73.

lat pull down, bicep curl, and leg curl), the deadlift took the longest to recuperate from (i.e., only 60% of the subjects were recovered by 48 hrs.).[294]

RECOVERY IS SPECIFIC TO EACH INDIVIDUAL

Recovery is required for adaptation to occur. If you examine the importance of recovery in both elite and amateur rugby players, both perceive recovery as equally important to enhance performance. However, elite Rugby athletes use significantly more recovery modalities (~8 vs. 3) than amateurs. Elite Rugby athletes implemented recovery modalities more often (~25 vs. ~6 times per week) compared to amateurs. Elite Rugby athletes perceived 6 out of 11 recovery modalities to be more effective than amateurs. Stretching, cold baths, active recovery, compression garments, massages, and pool recovery are the most used recovery modalities in the elite group with >90% of the athletes.[295] This is an example of elite athletes using more recovery methods than amateurs.

Many lifters don't enjoy taking time off; they want to train hard year-round. If you have performed a well-structured training cycle, you will look forward to a recovery phase! After recovery, a super-compensation period in which muscle growth will follow. For example, a 2019 study found that after two blocks of intense blood flow restriction training. In the initial five-day training block of intense exercise, there was a decrease in muscle size of Type I (-6%) and Type II (-16%) muscles fibers at baseline to Day 4. Then, a super-compensation phase took place after a 10-day rest period in which there was an increase in muscle growth of both Type I (+ 19%)

---

294 John A. Korak, James Matt Green, and Eric K. O'Neal, "Resistance Training Recovery: Considerations For Single Vs. Multi-Joint Movements And Upper Vs. Lower Body Muscles," *Medicine & Science in Sports & Exercise* 46 (May 2014): 193–94.

295 Francisco Tavares et al., "The Usage and Perceived Effectiveness of Different Recovery Modalities in Amateur and Elite Rugby Athletes," *Performance Enhancement & Health* 5, no. 4 (June 1, 2017): 142–46.

and Type II (+11%) muscles fibers.[296] This provides insight into a delayed super-compensation period in which muscle growth can overshoot after a period of intense exercise, followed by a recovery period.

The super-compensation model is the basis for resistance exercise-induced muscle growth. The first phase is the workout or alarm phase, which leads to a decline in one's "fitness" level (or performance). After the workout, the body starts recovering to reach the original "fitness" level (resistance phase). If recovery is adequate, then super-compensation occurs, increasing the "fitness" level above the original base.[297] It's essential for all people wishing to build muscle to include a *deload period* in their program to systematically reduce training volume and enhance recuperation. Other forms of recovery during a training day are taking light days to improve recovery and days off to rest the body completely. Recovery is dependent on several factors.[298] The critical defining list of general recovery features are:

- Recovery depends on the type of and duration of stress.

- Recovery depends on reducing stress, a change of stress, or a break from stress.

- Recovery is specific to the individual and depends on individual appraisal.

- Recovery can be passive, active, or pro-active.

- Recovery is closely tied to situational conditions.

296 Thomas Bjørnsen et al., ~Delayed Myonuclear Addition, Myofiber Hypertrophy, and Increases in Strength with High-Frequency Low-Load Blood Flow Restricted Training to Volitional Failure," *Journal of Applied Physiology (Bethesda, Md.: 1985)* 126, no. 3 (March 1, 2019): 578–92.

297 Janice S. Todd, Jason P. Shurley, and Terry C. Todd, "Thomas L. DeLorme and the Science of Progressive Resistance Exercise," *Journal of Strength and Conditioning Research* 26, no. 11 (November 2012): 2913–23.

298 M. Kellmann, "Preventing Overtraining in Athletes in High-Intensity Sports and Stress/Recovery Monitoring," *Scandinavian Journal of Medicine & Science in Sports* 20, no. s2 (2010): 95–102.

When most people read stress, they only think of stress created by a workout; however, mental stress can have a greater impact than exercise stress. A study found that athletes who were stressed out for personal reasons took longer to recuperate from exercise. Subjects who had little stress in their lives recuperated from exercise 24 hours after exercise, whereas those that had more mental stress recuperated 96 hours after exercise.[299] A study in mice found that creating psychological stress increased the muscle suppressing gene myostatin.[300] In a study of 135 college students assigned to a resistance exercise program to determine peak strength. Those who had low stress had greater increases in the bench press than those who had high stress.[301] It is important to remember that muscles grow during recovery. Too much stress, both mentally and physically, can hinder your muscle gains.

Taking rest days, strategic deloads in which the weight is reduced, active recovery with low-intensity exercise, and listening to your body are all critical for recovery. There are many new training devices, such as using heart rate variability (HRV) for monitoring fatigue and readiness to train. These devices are still debatable as to their effectiveness. One study found that HRV was not related to perceived recovery, muscle soreness, movement velocity, or vertical jump power.[302] More research needs to be

---

299 Matthew A. Stults-Kolehmainen, John B. Bartholomew, and Rajita Sinha, "Chronic Psychological Stress Impairs Recovery of Muscular Function and Somatic Sensations over a 96-Hour Period," *Journal of Strength and Conditioning Research* 28, no. 7 (July 2014): 2007–17.

300 David L. Allen et al., "Acute Daily Psychological Stress Causes Increased Atrophic Gene Expression and Myostatin-Dependent Muscle Atrophy," *American Journal of Physiology-Regulatory, Integrative and Comparative Physiology* 299, no. 3 (September 1, 2010): R889–98.

301 John B. Bartholomew et al., "Strength Gains after Resistance Training: The Effect of Stressful, Negative Life Events," *Journal of Strength and Conditioning Research* 22, no. 4 (July 2008): 1215–21.

302 Andrew A. Flatt et al., "Heart Rate Variability, Neuromuscular and Perceptual Recovery Following Resistance Training," *Sports (Basel, Switzerland)* 7, no. 10 (October 18, 2019): E225.

conducted before solely using heart rate variability devices as your sole method of recovery.

Deloads in which the total workout volume is systematically reduced for recovery should be taken every 4–6 weeks. During a deload, you reduce your training volume by 50% for a week to improve recovery and reduce fatigue. Remember, each of us has an individual recovery rate, and not everyone will recuperate the same. One fascinating case study was on an elite Olympic weightlifter who ranked top five in the world and was drug tested for anabolic steroids for the Olympics repeatedly. They documented his testosterone, IGF-1, and cortisol responses as the volume of his workouts increased. After the high-volume training, serum IGF-1, testosterone, and free testosterone decreased, whereas cortisol levels increased. *Even after the weightlifter tapered his volume workouts, free cortisol levels remained high after 6 weeks.* It indicated that the physiological stress induced by such training may last for more than 6 weeks, even when the training volume was markedly decreased by more than 50%.[303] This is just an example of someone needing an extended recovery time to reduce his cortisol levels after high volume training.

DELOADS

A deload is a planned reduction in workload to reduce training stress, drop fatigue, and give the nervous system a rest. Many lifters will train all year long without a break. In a survey of 605 competitive athletes, unexplained decreases in performance were reported by 71% of athletes, and 77% of these respondents were involved in resistance exercise-only sports. Acute maladaptation indicating acute fatigue was experienced by 71% of the

---

303 Ching-Lin Wu et al., "Hormonal Responses in Heavy Training and Recovery Periods in an Elite Male Weightlifter," *Journal of Sports Science & Medicine* 7 (December 1, 2008): 560–61.

athletes who reported an unexplained decrease in performance.[304] When the researchers further examined the reasons for training maladaptation, the following reasons were identified:

- Those with a greater resistance training age were not more likely to report unexplained decreases in performance.

- A large proportion of athletes reporting severe training maladaptation (>4 months) reported training to muscular failure.

- General feelings of fatigue were the most common self-reported symptom of acute and chronic maladaptation.

- Musculoskeletal aches and pains were the second most frequent self-reported symptom of acute maladaptation.

This survey indicates overtraining is more prevalent in the resistance training genre and that systemic fatigue is a primary indicator of overtraining. Other benefits of a deload are providing a psychological break, allowing for joint and connective tissue recovery, and potentially producing more muscle growth. Short-term deloads can result in greater increases in strength training.[305,306] Many lifters don't believe in taking breaks. Despite many people not wanting to rest, there are no negative consequences to taking a deload after a high-volume training mesocycle.

---

304 Clementine Grandou et al., "Symptoms of Overtraining in Resistance Exercise: International Cross-Sectional Survey," *International Journal of Sports Physiology and Performance* 16, no. 1 (July 17, 2020): 80–89.

305 M. J. Gibala, J. D. MacDougall, and D. G. Sale, "The Effects of Tapering on Strength Performance in Trained Athletes," *International Journal of Sports Medicine* 15, no. 8 (November 1994): 492–97.

306 Mikel Izquierdo et al., "Detraining and Tapering Effects on Hormonal Responses and Strength Performance," *Journal of Strength and Conditioning Research* 21, no. 3 (August 2007): 768–75.

WILL I LOSE MUSCLE DURING A DELOAD?

One of the biggest misconceptions is that if a person takes time off from the gym, they will lose muscle. Researchers had subjects that were divided into two groups. One group trained continuously over 24 weeks, whereas the other group performed periodic resistance training, in which they trained for six weeks and had a 3-week detraining period. This was repeated twice. At the end of the study, both groups had similar increases in strength and muscle size.[307] If you do a thorough analysis of the study, the group that took off the 3 weeks had initial losses in strength and size, but this was regained rapidly when training resumed. The retraining group gained muscle twice as fast as that of the continuous group, so by the end of each 6-week retraining phase, the periodic group had caught up with the continuous group. In another study, resistance-trained men followed a 4-day per week program in which they trained for 4 weeks, did not train for 2 weeks, and then re-trained again for another 4 weeks. When they stopped training for two weeks, there was no decrease in muscle mass or strength (lean mass was retained); when they retrained, muscle mass increased.[308] Other studies have shown that deloads for 3–5 days can reduce fatigue, increase strength, and increase muscle size.[309,310]

What if you are the type of person who can't take off? You want to do some exercise but keep it light weight. Researchers compared active vs.

---

307 Riki Ogasawara et al., "Comparison of Muscle Hypertrophy Following 6-Month of Continuous and Periodic Strength Training," *European Journal of Applied Physiology* 113, no. 4 (April 2013): 975–85.

308 Paul S. Hwang et al., "Resistance Training-Induced Elevations in Muscular Strength in Trained Men Are Maintained After 2 Weeks of Detraining and Not Differentially Affected by Whey Protein Supplementation," *Journal of Strength and Conditioning Research* 31, no. 4 (April 2017): 869–81.

309 Hayden J. Pritchard et al., "Short-Term Training Cessation as a Method of Tapering to Improve Maximal Strength," *Journal of Strength and Conditioning Research* 32, no. 2 (February 2018): 458–65.

310 Hagen Hartmann et al., "Short-Term Periodization Models: Effects on Strength and Speed-Strength Performance," *Sports Medicine (Auckland, N.Z.)* 45, no. 10 (October 2015): 1373–86.

passive recovery after an intense 6-week protocol during which, in the final week, they were using 32 sets per body part. The passive recovery group stopped training, whereas the active recovery group had a deload of 85% reduction in volume (5 sets per week). At the end of the study, there was no difference in muscle mass, anabolic signaling pathways, cortisol, etc. So, you can either drop your volume significantly or take a week off; both are completely fine, depending on your preference.[311] Another study found that when subjects went from training with an excess of 20+ sets and then cut sets back to 8 sets, they maintained muscle size.[312]

If you are dealing with external emotional stress, muscle gains can also be compromised. If you are a serious athlete and training hard, deloads are essential for making new gains in muscle and strength. Some of the biggest concerns with lifters about why they won't take a deload are: they think they will lose muscle and strength. These concerns are not warranted during a short-term deload.

If you are going to keep training during a deload, here are some general tips:

- Cut back on volume dramatically (50% reduction)

- Cut back on the weight you normally would use 40-50%

- Cut back on training to failure with 5 RIR.

- Slowly increase volume once you resume training. Don't jump back to your previous training volume.

*A deload should be added to your routine every 4–8 weeks, depending on your fatigue levels.

---

311 Christopher G. Vann et al., "Molecular Differences in Skeletal Muscle After 1 Week of Active vs. Passive Recovery From High volume Resistance Training," *Journal of Strength and Conditioning Research* 35, no. 8 (August 1, 2021): 2102–13.

312 Lucas Duarte Tavares et al., "Effects of Different Strength Training Frequencies during Reduced Training Period on Strength and Muscle Cross-Sectional Area," *European Journal of Sport Science* 17, no. 6 (July 2017): 665–72.

STARTING A NEW PROGRAM CYCLE

When you start a new training cycle after a deload and have dropped your volume, consider changing all the exercises if your primary goal is muscle growth. It's very important to know that you will be very sore once you start a new exercise routine! Why? Remember, the repeated bout effect takes place over a period of weeks to protect your muscles from further damage. Training a muscle from a new angle (i.e., unaccustomed exercise) is a new stressor for your body to adapt to. Also, your RIR should be in the 4–5 range your first week back from a deload and gradually decrease your RIR as your volume increases over the mesocycle.

MUSCLEGATE: ICE BATHS ENHANCE RECOVERY AND MUSCLE GROWTH

THE TRUTH EXPOSED: Cryotherapy and ice baths are the rage today for recuperation. They all point to reducing inflammation, reducing muscle soreness, and improving recovery.[313] The use of cold-water therapy is not without drawbacks; some studies have found no benefit in using cold water immersion post-exercise to reduce muscle soreness.[314,315] Others have found that cold water immersion long-term (16 weeks) can reduce muscle growth! Subjects performed an intense resistance training protocol, and either sat in an ice bath for 10 minutes or performed an active recovery. The investigators found that cold water immersion blunted

---

313 Chris Bleakley et al., "Cold-Water Immersion (Cryotherapy) for Preventing and Treating Muscle Soreness after Exercise," *The Cochrane Database of Systematic Reviews*, no. 2 (February 15, 2012): CD008262.

314 Pinto, J., Rocha, P., & Torres, R. (2020). Cold-Water Immersion Has No Effect on Muscle Stiffness After Exercise-Induced Muscle Damage. Clinical journal of sport medicine : official journal of the Canadian Academy of Sport Medicine, 30(6), 533–538.

315 Jonathan M. Peake et al., "The Effects of Cold Water Immersion and Active Recovery on Inflammation and Cell Stress Responses in Human Skeletal Muscle after Resistance Exercise," *The Journal of Physiology* 595, no. 3 (February 1, 2017): 695–711.

anabolic signaling pathways and reduced strength and muscle growth.[316,317] In a review of effective recovery modalities, massage, compression garments, and cold-water immersion are the most effective recovery modalities. Massage has the most beneficial effect on muscle soreness and fatigue. Although, to a lesser extent, compression garments and cold-water immersion also have a beneficial effect on both muscle soreness and fatigue. Cold modalities (e.g., cryotherapy and cold-water immersion) and massage elicit the greatest effects on reducing muscle damage markers.[318] Inflammation is part of the normal healing process; cryotherapy, cold water immersion, and ibuprofen block the normal inflammation process and reduces muscle growth. Non-steroidal anti-inflammatory drugs (NSAIDs) and anti-inflammatories blunt the adaptation responses for muscle growth to occur. Research has shown that taking ibuprofen and other NSAIDS can reduce muscle protein synthesis and reduce muscle growth.[319] Stay away from NSAIDs like the plague if you are trying to gain muscle.

316 Llion A. Roberts et al., "Post-Exercise Cold Water Immersion Attenuates Acute Anabolic Signalling and Long-Term Adaptations in Muscle to Strength Training," *The Journal of Physiology* 593, no. 18 (2015): 4285–4301.

317 Jackson J. Fyfe et al., "Cold Water Immersion Attenuates Anabolic Signaling and Skeletal Muscle Fiber Hypertrophy, but Not Strength Gain, Following Whole-Body Resistance Training," *Journal of Applied Physiology (Bethesda, Md.: 1985)* 127, no. 5 (November 1, 2019): 1403–18.

318 Olivier Dupuy et al., "An Evidence-Based Approach for Choosing Post-Exercise Recovery Techniques to Reduce Markers of Muscle Damage, Soreness, Fatigue, and Inflammation: A Systematic Review With Meta-Analysis," *Frontiers in Physiology* 9 (2018): 403.

319 Tommy R. Lundberg and Glyn Howatson, "Analgesic and Anti-Inflammatory Drugs in Sports: Implications for Exercise Performance and Training Adaptations," *Scandinavian Journal of Medicine & Science in Sports* 28, no. 11 (November 2018): 2252–62.

CHAPTER SUMMARY:

- There are two types of fatigue: Central fatigue (brain) and peripheral fatigue (muscle).

- Compound movements can cause greater central fatigue than single-joint exercises.

- Athletes with more Type II fibers experience greater fatigue and are more likely to overtrain with high volume.

- Building muscle is highly individualized; some people recover faster and slower than others.

- Deloads are essential for reducing fatigue, enhancing recovery, and allowing for super-compensation.

- Cold water therapy and NSAIDS are not conducive for muscle growth.

CHAPTER 9

REST PERIODS

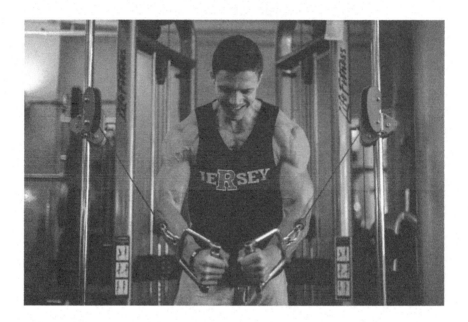

For the past decade, bodybuilders have been training with 60 second rest periods to boost metabolic stress and elicit greater anabolic hormones. Using short rest periods results in a greater physiological and perceptual response than taking longer rest periods. New research suggests that shorter rest periods may not be the best approach for building muscle.

MUSCLEGATE: SHORT REST PERIODS PROMOTE MUSCLE GROWTH

THE TRUTH EXPOSED: One of the other biggest myths is that increased metabolic stress by taking short rest periods results in more muscle growth. This is why people incorporate techniques like supersets and drop-sets and use short rest periods to increase lactate and metabolic stress. In the coolest study of the year, researchers infused lactate in the bloodstream of resistance-trained men. Post-exercise, the subjects that had the infusion had higher blood lactate levels. Still, they did not have any additional increases in protein synthesis compared to the regular resistance exercise group. This dispels the myth that metabolic stress (increased lactate) has some magical muscle-promoting effect.[320] Other studies have reported that short rest periods (1 minute), despite higher lactate, resulted in less protein synthesis (68%) post-exercise, compared to 5 minutes (139%).[321] Another study found that comparing 30-second rest periods to 150-second rest periods using the same total workload resulted in similar muscle growth. Still, greater muscle growth trended towards the group that took longer rest periods.[322] Note that smaller muscle groups like the abs, calves, and arms can be trained with shorter rest periods, while other muscle groups such as the quads, back, and chest will require longer rest periods. The major drawback of taking short rest periods is that you begin sets fatigued, which results in less total volume. Volume is a potent stimulator of muscle growth to a certain point. By using short rest periods, each

---

320 Rasmus Liegnell et al., "Elevated Plasma Lactate Levels via Exogenous Lactate Infusion Do Not Alter Resistance Exercise-Induced Signaling or Protein Synthesis in Human Skeletal Muscle," *American Journal of Physiology. Endocrinology and Metabolism* 319, no. 4 (October 1, 2020): E792–804.

321 James McKendry et al., "Short Inter-Set Rest Blunts Resistance Exercise-Induced Increases in Myofibrillar Protein Synthesis and Intracellular Signalling in Young Males," *Experimental Physiology* 101, no. 7 (July 1, 2016): 866–82.

322 Julius Etienne Fink et al., "Acute and Long-Term Responses to Different Rest Intervals in Low-Load Resistance Training," *International Journal of Sports Medicine* 38, no. 2 (February 2017): 118–24.

additional set will lead to a reduction in repetitions, resulting in a reduced total workload volume.

If metabolic stress were the primary driver of muscle growth, then eccentric exercise would cause very little muscle growth because metabolically eccentric contractions produce very little metabolic stress. Studies have found that eccentric exercise produces less metabolic stress (i.e., lactate) compared with concentric exercise. The metabolic cost required for eccentric exercise is approximately fourfold lower than for the same exercise performed concentrically. Reduced cardiorespiratory and hemodynamic responses have been reported following eccentric exercise compared to concentric exercise at the same absolute workload.[323] However, eccentric exercise still contributes to muscle growth, despite less metabolic stress. When concentric and eccentric exercises are performed at the same absolute workload, similar increases in muscle growth occur, despite lower metabolic stress occurring with eccentric exercises.[324] Also, there are *blood flow restriction* programs in which pressure is applied with a tourniquet around the legs. This generates high metabolic stress because of hypoxia (absence of oxygen). When comparing studies that use tourniquet training or blood flow restriction training with weights compared to blood flow restriction training without weight (i.e., researchers applied blood flow restriction but no exercise), both produce metabolic stress. However, only the group that performed tourniquet training with weights experienced increased muscle protein synthesis and muscle growth.[325] Metabolic stress must be combined with tension for muscle growth to occur. It's more likely that muscle tension, not metabolic stress, is driving muscle growth. There

323 T. J. Overend et al., "Cardiovascular Stress Associated with Concentric and Eccentric Isokinetic Exercise in Young and Older Adults," *The Journals of Gerontology. Series A, Biological Sciences and Medical Sciences* 55, no. 4 (April 2000): B177-182.

324 Martino V. Franchi, Neil D. Reeves, and Marco V. Narici, "Skeletal Muscle Remodeling in Response to Eccentric vs. Concentric Loading: Morphological, Molecular, and Metabolic Adaptations," *Frontiers in Physiology* 8 (July 4, 2017): 447.

325 JEAN NYAKAYIRU et al., "Blood Flow Restriction Only Increases Myofibrillar Protein Synthesis with Exercise," *Medicine and Science in Sports and Exercise* 51, no. 6 (June 2019): 1137–45.

is intense debate whether metabolic stress is a driving factor for muscle growth, but more research needs to be conducted.

MUSCLEGATE: TAKING 1-MINUTE REST PERIODS BOOSTS MUSCLE GROWTH

THE TRUTH EXPOSED: Back in the early 90s, several studies came out and showed that men who performed bodybuilding style routines (10–12 reps) with 1-minute rest periods produced greater growth hormone (GH) testosterone than powerlifters lifting with 3-minute rest periods.[326] This led to a rise in all bodybuilders taking short rest periods to get the greatest anabolic hormone levels during their workout. As you have read previously, acute anabolic hormone responses have little impact on muscle growth. Short rest periods reduce the quality of effective reps because they must use less weight/reps and, therefore, less tension on the muscle. Shorter rest periods mean you will perform fewer repetitions than the previous set, resulting in lower training volume. *Longer rest periods have been found to result in greater muscle growth!* I know I am killing a decade of bodybuilding magazines that promote the *Short Rest Periods for Size*, but the truth hurts. Short rest periods will result in a greater muscle pump due to greater metabolic stress, which will not lead to greater muscle growth. In 2016, muscle guru Ph.D. Brad Schoenfeld found that *lifters who used a 3-minute rest period had greater muscle growth than groups using 1-minute rest periods.*[327] A similar study found that training with 1-minute rest periods resulted in roughly half the muscle growth compared to a

326 William J. Kraemer and Nicholas A. Ratamess, "Hormonal Responses and Adaptations to Resistance Exercise and Training," *Sports Medicine (Auckland, N.Z.)* 35, no. 4 (2005): 339–61.

327 Brad J. Schoenfeld et al., "Longer Interset Rest Periods Enhance Muscle Strength and Hypertrophy in Resistance-Trained Men," *Journal of Strength and Conditioning Research* 30, no. 7 (July 2016): 1805–12.

3-minute rest period.[328] Another big problem with short rest periods is that it severely limits the weight you can lift the next set. By resting longer, you will use the same weight and do more repetitions the next set, resulting in a greater training volume. Heavy weight resistance exercise seems to provide a superior muscle growth response to light weight training not taken to complete failure. Heavy weight provides a greater muscle growth stimulus for all muscle fibers.[329] You may want to ditch the stopwatch and use your perception of whether you are ready to do a set. Researchers found that when subjects were told to "Choose a rest period you feel will allow you to complete a maximal effort during your next set" while doing a heavy squat protocol of 5 sets for 5 reps; nearly 100% of the subjects completed all the prescribed sets and reps successfully.[330] The rest times averaged between 4 and 5 minutes, but again this was using a powerlifting type protocol, but for bodybuilders, the research recommends greater than 3 minutes rest periods for muscle growth. Rest periods are subjective. Perform your next set when you feel that you have fully recovered from the previous set for optimal muscle growth.

The biggest issue with short rest periods is that you begin your next set in a fatigued state, which leads to a diminished training volume. The other issue with short rest periods with large muscle groups like the legs will result in a massive cardiovascular demand! You will breathe like a freight train after 1-minute rest periods with squats. Before starting your next set, ask yourself, has my breathing returned to normal? You are training to build muscle, not get a cardiovascular workout! Also, is a synergistic muscle used in the exercise still fatigued? For example, are your triceps still

---

328 Ariel Roberth Longo et al., "Volume Load Rather Than Resting Interval Influences Muscle Hypertrophy During High-Intensity Resistance Training," *The Journal of Strength & Conditioning Research*, 9000.

329 Jozo Grgic and Brad J. Schoenfeld, "Are the Hypertrophic Adaptations to High and Low-Load Resistance Training Muscle Fiber Type Specific?," *Frontiers in Physiology* 9 (April 18, 2018): 402.

330 P. Ibbott et al., "Variability and Impact of Self-Selected Interset Rest Periods During Experienced Strength Training," *Perceptual and Motor Skills* 126, no. 3 (June 2019): 546–58.

burning from your last set of bench presses? If you start your next set with pre-fatigued triceps, your training volume for the chest will go down.

SHORT REST PERIODS: MORE SETS FOR THE SAME RESULTS

The problem with comparing short versus longer rest periods studies is that the longer rest period groups can do more volume (sets x reps). What if you had the short rest period do more sets to equate the volume from longer rest periods? Would it build more muscle? Researchers had subjects train for 10 weeks, but they equated the volume of longer rest periods by having the 1-minute group do more sets until the total volume was similar. When the volume was equated, both the short rest period and longer rest period group had similar increases in muscle growth; however, *the short rest period group had to do 50% more sets to compensate for the reduced volume that the longer rest period group completed!*[331] The big question is, "Why would anyone want to perform double the sets when you can achieve the same results with longer rest periods?" In a 2018 meta-analysis of rest period durations, 23 studies comprising 491 participants (413 males and 78 females) were analyzed. Results of the literature review found that significant gains in strength can be achieved even with short rest periods of less than <60 seconds. *However, longer duration rest intervals (>2 min) are needed to maximize strength gains in resistance-trained individuals, whereas short to moderate rest intervals (60–120 s) are sufficient for maximizing muscular strength gains in untrained individuals.*[332] This suggests that taking longer rest periods will maximize muscle strength gains and muscle growth. ***One should rest until they are ready to perform their next set,***

331 Ariel Roberth Longo et al., "Volume Load Rather Than Resting Interval Influences Muscle Hypertrophy During High-Intensity Resistance Training," *The Journal of Strength & Conditioning Research*, October 7, 2021.

332 Jozo Grgic et al., "Effects of Rest Interval Duration in Resistance Training on Measures of Muscular Strength: A Systematic Review," *Sports Medicine (Auckland, N.Z.)* 48, no. 1 (January 2018): 137–51.

and it should not be determined by a clock. In some muscle groups like the arms and calves, you can probably use 1 minute rest periods and perform the next set. Exercises that incorporate a large number of muscle groups like deadlifts and squats will require longer rest periods to maximize volume and muscle hypertrophy.

ACUTE ANABOLIC HORMONES
DON'T BUILD MUSCLE

What about the acute increases in hormones? Short rest periods increase GH and testosterone more than longer rest periods. A landmark study had subjects use the same total workout volume (reps x sets x weight lifted) but different rest periods between sets (2 min vs. 5 min). The cool thing about this study was that it was a six-month crossover design in two 3-month block sessions. Half of the participants trained using 2-minute rest intervals between sets for the first block, and the other half trained using 5-minute rest intervals between sets. At the end of the six months, there was no significant difference between testosterone, free testosterone, or GH between the short and long rest period groups. *Also, both groups had similar gains in muscle mass and strength.*[333] This suggests that you can rest anywhere between 2-5 minutes between sets and obtain similar results based on your preference. Multi-joint exercises like the squat, deadlift, clean and jerk, etc., will require 2–5-minute rest between sets, but isolation exercises like the curls and calf raises can be exercised with shorter rest periods.

If you are using the latest technology to boost muscle growth, you may want to incorporate some blood flow restriction (BFR) training into your routine. Please make sure you have an experienced coach assisting you with BFR. Researchers had subjects complete seven sets (two-minutes

---

333 Juha P. Ahtiainen et al., "Short vs. Long Rest Period between the Sets in Hypertrophic Resistance Training: Influence on Muscle Strength, Size, and Hormonal Adaptations in Trained Men," *Journal of Strength and Conditioning Research* 19, no. 3 (August 2005): 572–82.

rest between sets) with 10 repetitions of back squatting at 70% of 1RM. During the two-minute rest period, the right leg had a BFR cuff inflated to a pressure of 230 mmHg, whereas the left leg served as a control. They did not exercise and only had a BFR cuff inflated to max capacity on one leg during rest periods. Muscle biopsies were taken on both legs two hours after the workout session. There were different responses with the leg that had the BFR cuff inflated between rest periods. Resistance exercise with BFR used between rest periods increased key signaling proteins involved in protein synthesis, vascularization, mitochondrial biogenesis, and the antioxidant system. Also, BFR increased genes related to muscle damage and repair that were not increased with the control leg.[334] This was a very small study, but it's promising to show that using BFR in the rest periods without exercises can increase muscle hypertrophy. It should be mentioned that there are some very effective training strategies, such as cluster set training, which incorporate short rest periods and enhance muscle mass; this will be discussed in Chapter 14.

Keep in mind that the acute changes in testosterone that typically occur with short rest periods *last for about an hour* and then return to baseline quickly. Many lifters like to compare the acute anabolic hormone increases after exercise to pharmacological increases in testosterone. If you compare the dosage response of low-dose testosterone replacement therapy, there is a sustained release in testosterone *over several hours.*[335] Acute anabolic *may* contribute to muscle growth but based on the research, it is relatively small.

---

334 Ferenc Torma et al., "Blood Flow Restriction in Human Skeletal Muscle during Rest Periods after High-Load Resistance Training down-Regulates MiR-206 and Induces Pax7," *Journal of Sport and Health Science* 10, no. 4 (July 1, 2021): 470–77.

335 A. S. Dobs et al., "Pharmacokinetics, Efficacy, and Safety of a Permeation-Enhanced Testosterone Transdermal System in Comparison with Bi-Weekly Injections of Testosterone Enanthate for the Treatment of Hypogonadal Men," *The Journal of Clinical Endocrinology and Metabolism* 84, no. 10 (October 1999): 3469–78.

VOLUME INCREASES MUSCLE GROWTH

Remember, in the previous chapters, I discussed a positive relationship between volume and muscle growth. Volume goes down with short rest periods; you need to reduce the weight to compensate for the fatigue by resting less. When researchers used various rest periods and determined their effect on volume, short rest periods resulted in the shortest workout volume. Subjects performed the bench press in the 5–10 rep range. The rest intervals were: 30 seconds, 1 minute, 2 minutes, 3 minutes, and 5 minutes. The largest reductions in performance occurred with very short rest (<1 min), and performance was maintained during the first 3-4 sets when 3 – and 5-min rest intervals were used.[336] This suggests that longer rest periods enable a larger work volume during exercise. Longer rest periods between sets reduce fatigue and enable you to regenerate more ATP (i.e., the body's energy currency) for high-intensity exercise.

FLEXING BETWEEN SETS TO GAIN MORE MUSCLE?

Here is a training tip. Squeezing the muscle or an isometric contraction between sets during your rest period *may* enhance muscle growth after compound movements. It's well known that bodybuilders will spend hours practicing their posing routine in front of the mirror before a show to make sure their posing presentation is flawless. If you have ever watched a posing routine, it's not exactly easy; hitting isometric poses often can leave a bodybuilder exhausted. Some bodybuilders even swear it helps build muscle prepping for a show. In 2014, Maeo et al. provided some research that validated these beliefs. He had subjects squeeze their biceps and triceps simultaneously as hard as they could for four seconds for 12 weeks without any external resistance (i.e., no weight). At the end of 12 weeks,

---

336 Nicholas A. Ratamess et al., "The Effect of Rest Interval Length on Metabolic Responses to the Bench Press Exercise.," *European Journal of Applied Physiology* 100, no. 1 (May 2007): 1–17.

the subjects had a 4% increase in muscle growth of the biceps and triceps *without any external resistance.*[337] This suggests that isometric contractions can enhance muscle growth. A follow-up investigation in 2020 found similar benefits for squeezing the muscle as hard as you can to build muscle in conjunction with resistance exercise. Researchers found that when subjects contracted the muscle, they were exercising between sets; they tended to have greater muscle growth in only the legs. In contrast, other body parts such as the biceps and triceps, were not affected compared to those that rested.[338] Subjects held a five-second isometric contraction or, in layman's terms, flexed at the end of each set. Isometric contractions are something you can add to your training while you are resting between sets that may squeeze out a little more muscle growth. Another technique to use during rest periods is shaking your muscles and relaxing them. Some lifters had small improvements in strength when they shook the muscles for 30 seconds between exercises.[339] Consider incorporating some muscle-flexing between sets while you are resting.

---

337 Sumiaki Maeo et al., "Neuromuscular Adaptations Following 12-Week Maximal Voluntary Co-Contraction Training," *European Journal of Applied Physiology* 114, no. 4 (April 1, 2014): 663–73.

338 Brad J. Schoenfeld et al., "To Flex or Rest: Does Adding No-Load Isometric Actions to the Inter-Set Rest Period in Resistance Training Enhance Muscular Adaptations? A Randomized-Controlled Trial," *Frontiers in Physiology* 10 (2020): 1571.

339 Brendan L. Pinto and Stuart M. McGill, "Voluntary Muscle Relaxation Can Mitigate Fatigue and Improve Countermovement Jump Performance," *Journal of Strength and Conditioning Research* 34, no. 6 (June 2020): 1525–29.

CHAPTER SUMMARY:

- Longer rest periods have been found to result in greater muscle growth!

- Short rest periods severely limit the weight you can lift the next set and reduce training volume.

- Short rest periods can be beneficial for isolation exercises such as preacher curls, triceps extension, etc.

- Multi-joint exercises require longer rest periods.

CHAPTER 10:
TRAINING FREQUENCY

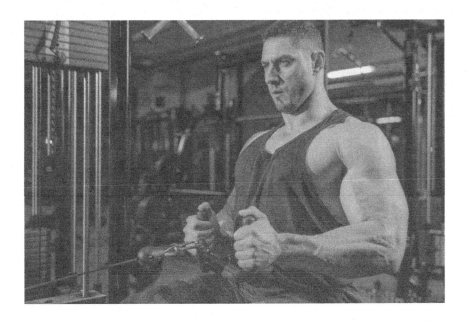

Training frequency is often a topic of conversation for increasing muscle growth. Is it better to train a muscle once, twice, or even three times a week? Most bodybuilders will break their workouts into splits, so they will do a major body part such as the chest and combine it with a smaller bodypart such as the triceps. Others will work their entire body in one workout. Another popular topic is training twice per day (morning and evening sessions). By breaking your workout into morning and evening sessions, the theory is that greater protein synthesis and anabolic hormones will be stimulated than one workout per day, leading to greater increases in muscle growth.

MUSCLEGATE: TRAINING EACH MUSCLE GROUP ONCE A WEEK MAXIMIZES MUSCLE GROWTH

THE TRUTH EXPOSED: A 2013 survey reported that 70% of the bodybuilders trained each body part once per week, whereas 31% trained each muscle group twice per week.[340] Going to the gym stimulates muscle growth by causing tension to muscle fibers, followed by recuperation and muscle protein synthesis.

Beginner's experience much more damage to exercise than trained athletes. If you are a beginner, once-a-week training is sufficient to stimulate muscle growth. Still, as you continue to train, your body adapts to the exercise program and becomes more resilient to muscle damage. This process of muscle adaptations to exercise is called the *repeated bout effect*.[341] The ability to train a muscle group again is determined by whether you have recuperated from your previous exercise bout. Your ability to train a muscle again depends on your genetic ability to recuperate (i.e., number of Type II fibers), which muscle group is being trained (i.e., calves can be trained more often than hamstrings), and the type of workout (i.e., an eccentric overload program will take longer to recuperate between workouts than a traditional resistance exercise protocol).

Trained athletes have less of an increase in muscle protein synthesis and less muscle damage after exercise than untrained athletes, which means trained athletes need more training stimulus to keep building muscle.[342] If you train a muscle group once a week and the muscle has recuperated, waiting an additional week will result in subpar muscle gains. It should also

---

340 Daniel A. Hackett, Nathan A. Johnson, and Chin-Moi Chow, "Training Practices and Ergogenic Aids Used by Male Bodybuilders," *Journal of Strength and Conditioning Research* 27, no. 6 (June 2013): 1609–17.

341 Robert D. Hyldahl, Trevor C. Chen, and Kazunori Nosaka, "Mechanisms and Mediators of the Skeletal Muscle Repeated Bout Effect," *Exercise and Sport Sciences Reviews* 45, no. 1 (January 2017): 24–33.

342 Felipe Damas et al., "A Review of Resistance Training-Induced Changes in Skeletal Muscle Protein Synthesis and Their Contribution to Hypertrophy," *Sports Medicine (Auckland, N.Z.)* 45, no. 6 (June 2015): 801–7.

be mentioned that after 10 weeks of resistance exercise, untrained athletes also have a dampening of muscle protein synthesis.[343] This shows that after 10 weeks, they have reached an adaptation process.

If you examine the studies regarding training frequency, *training a muscle group twice a week was superior to training a muscle group once a week for muscle growth.*[344] Other studies found that greater training frequency resulted in greater muscle mass independent of training volume.[345] What if we decide to increase the frequency even more? Does that translate into more muscle growth? One study compared training with 4 sessions per week, 4 days (Mondays, Tuesdays, Thursdays, and Fridays) to twice per week (Mondays and Thursdays). The twice per week sessions were a high-volume session, low frequency (36 sets per workout), whereas the four days per week were high frequency but low volume (18 sets per workout). There was no difference between lean mass and strength gains after six weeks between the groups for the legs, but the high frequency (4 days a week) had greater increases in upper body growth.[346] *This suggests that higher frequency training results in greater muscle growth.* There seems to be a threshold in which more frequent training is not beneficial. The use of high-frequency, low-volume sessions to stimulate muscle growth is called *micro-dosing.* It is the assumption that small frequent increases in protein synthesis and anabolic signaling pathways can possibly result in a larger muscle growth response. There are mixed results regarding the optimal frequency, as more does not always result in greater muscle growth. For

---

343 Felipe Damas et al., "Resistance Training-Induced Changes in Integrated Myofibrillar Protein Synthesis Are Related to Hypertrophy Only after Attenuation of Muscle Damage," *The Journal of Physiology* 594, no. 18 (September 15, 2016): 5209–22.

344 Brad J. Schoenfeld, Dan Ogborn, and James W. Krieger, "Effects of Resistance Training Frequency on Measures of Muscle Hypertrophy: A Systematic Review and Meta-Analysis," *Sports Medicine (Auckland, N.Z.)* 46, no. 11 (November 2016): 1689–97.

345 "Training Frequency for Strength Development: What the Data Say," *Stronger by Science* (blog), July 30, 2018,.

346 Fu Leon Yue et al., "Comparison of 2 Weekly-Equalized Volume Resistance-Training Routines Using Different Frequencies on Body Composition and Performance in Trained Males," *Applied Physiology, Nutrition, and Metabolism = Physiologie Appliquee, Nutrition Et Metabolisme* 43, no. 5 (May 2018): 475–81.

example, training six days a week results in no greater strength and muscle growth than three days a week.[347] A Canadian study found that training 2 days per week vs. 3 days a week resulted in similar muscle growth when the volume of resistance exercise was similar between the groups.[348] Whether you decide to do a full-body workout or perform a workout split, as long as the total volume is similar, both will equally increase muscle mass the same.[349] The advantage of adding frequency or extra days is that it is often difficult to add extra sets in a single session without fatigue. Increased frequency with the use of a whole-body workout training each muscle group three days a week resulted in greater muscle growth than the typical bodybuilding split, training each muscle group once a week.[350]

In 2017, an article titled, "Frequency: The Overlooked Resistance Training Variable for Inducing Muscle Hypertrophy?" suggests the following benefits for increasing working frequency: a.) Trained individuals should train similar muscle groups more frequently while reducing the number of sets performed in each training session. This is based on earlier research suggesting increasing the number of sets beyond a certain point has negligible effects on muscle hypertrophy, given the relatively low volume appears to maximally stimulate muscle protein synthesis; b) The duration of the time when muscle protein synthesis is elevated in trained individuals appears to be shortened. The authors of the study hypothesized that increasing training frequency, rather than training load or sets

347 Ryan J. Colquhoun et al., "Training Volume, Not Frequency, Indicative of Maximal Strength Adaptations to Resistance Training," *Journal of Strength and Conditioning Research* 32, no. 5 (May 2018): 1207–13.

348 Darren G. Candow and Darren G. Burke, "Effect of Short-Term Equal-Volume Resistance Training with Different Workout Frequency on Muscle Mass and Strength in Untrained Men and Women," *Journal of Strength and Conditioning Research* 21, no. 1 (February 2007): 204–7.

349 Alexandre Lopes Evangelista et al., "Split or Full-Body Workout Routine: Which Is Best to Increase Muscle Strength and Hypertrophy?," *Einstein (Sao Paulo, Brazil)* 19 (2021): eAO5781.

350 Brad J. Schoenfeld et al., "Influence of Resistance Training Frequency on Muscular Adaptations in Well-Trained Men," *The Journal of Strength & Conditioning Research* 29, no. 7 (July 2015): 1821–29.

performed, maybe a more effective strategy for trained individuals to increase muscle size.[351] An exciting abstract titled "Norwegian Frequency Project" found that increased training frequency was advantageous. Elite competitive Norwegian powerlifters were divided into two groups. One group trained 3 days per week, while another group trained 6 days per week. Both groups performed the resistance training program for 15 weeks using the same exercises, weekly volume, and intensity. At the end of the study, the 6 weekly training sessions, which used shorter but more frequent workouts, gained more strength and muscle mass than the 3 days per week group. The average increase in muscle mass for the 6 days per week group was almost 10% in the vastus lateralis and nearly 5% in the quadriceps.[352] Keep in mind that this was just an abstract and has never gone through the peer-review process.

The typical bodybuilders hit each body part once per week. It's smarter to break a workout into two parts and space them over the week than try to do it all in one day. For example, you will get a more effective workout if you break a chest workout into 8 sets on Monday and 8 sets on Friday instead of doing 16 sets all on Monday. After the first 5 sets, an enormous amount of fatigue can diminish the workout quality, leading to a reduced training volume. In a study on female athletes, increased muscle size was found when the total resistance training volume was split into two sessions per day instead of one. This suggests that distributing the volume of a resistance exercise program into smaller units, such as two daily sessions, may create more optimal conditions not only for muscular

---

351 Scott J. Dankel et al., "Frequency: The Overlooked Resistance Training Variable for Inducing Muscle Hypertrophy?," *Sports Medicine* 47, no. 5 (May 1, 2017): 799–805.

352 "Raastad T, Kirketeig, A, Wolf, D, Paulsen G. Powerlifters Improved Strength and Muscular Adaptations to a Greater Extent When Equal Total Training Volume Was Divided into 6 Compared to 3 Training Sessions per Week (Abstract). Book of Abstracts, 17th Annual Conference of the ECSS, Brugge 4-7 July, 2012.," n.d.

hypertrophy but by producing effective training stimuli, especially for the nervous system.[353]

It's recommended that you perform anywhere from 6–8 hard sets per body part each session. It's been found that 4 sets taken to complete muscular failure took 48 hours for complete muscle recovery to take place.[354] This suggests that the standard bodybuilding practice of training a muscle once per week is sub-par for increasing muscle growth for advanced trainers.

SUMMARY: There is no added benefit to increasing workout frequency per muscle group greater than 2–3 days a week. Total volume seems to be the determining factor for muscle growth rather than training frequency. If you do 20 sets per week, it does not seem to matter whether it's done in 2 sessions of 10 sets or 4 sessions with 5 sets. The driving factor for increasing workout frequency is to increase weekly total workout volume per bodypart.

MUSCLEGATE: TRAIN EVERY OTHER DAY TO BOOST MUSCLE GROWTH.

THE TRUTH EXPOSED: Muscle protein synthesis and repair occur after exercise, not during exercise. Logic dictates that having a day of recovery after an intense exercise session would facilitate muscle growth. Although this seems logical, science does not support this. Researchers compared lifters that did the same workout, trained to failure, used the same rest periods, and the same volume. The only difference was that one group trained consistently for 3 days in a row (~24 hours between sessions), whereas another group had a rest day after each workout (~48–72

---

353 K. Häkkinen and M. Kallinen, "Distribution of Strength Training Volume into One or Two Daily Sessions and Neuromuscular Adaptations in Female Athletes," *Electromyography and Clinical Neurophysiology* 34, no. 2 (March 1994): 117–24.

354 G. A. Paz et al., "Muscle Activation and Volume Load Performance of Paired Resistance Training Bouts with Differing Inter-Session Recovery Periods," *Science & Sports* 36, no. 2 (April 1, 2021): 152–59.

hours between sessions) for 12 weeks. At the end of the study, both groups had similar increases in muscle growth and strength.[355] When all training variables, such as volume, intensity, rest periods, etc., are equated, there does not seem to be a difference in whether you train 3 days in a row or space it out over the week.

MUSCLEGATE: TRAINING TWICE PER DAY FOR MORE MUSCLE GROWTH

THE TRUTH EXPOSED: Training twice a day does not increase muscle growth compared to once a day when the volume is similar between groups. Twice per day training could result in greater increases in anabolic hormones, leading to greater increases in muscle protein synthesis and anabolic signaling pathways. The rationale was that if resistance exercise provides an anabolic response, breaking sessions into two smaller sessions over the day could provide a greater stimulus for muscle growth. *If you examine the studies regarding muscle protein synthesis, volume seems to be the driving factor; not the frequency.*

For example, research had subjects perform 10 sets of leg exercises consisting of leg presses and leg extension *once per week*. The other group did the same exercises *every day* for 5 days (1 set of 10 reps for leg press and extensions). Thus, the weekly set volume was 10 sets total in both conditions; they performed it once or spread it across multiple days. At the end of the study, muscle protein synthesis and anabolic signaling pathways were the same between the groups.[356] The author concluded that when the volume is similar, training frequency does not impact protein synthesis.

---

355 Yifan Yang et al., "Effects of Consecutive Versus Non-Consecutive Days of Resistance Training on Strength, Body Composition, and Red Blood Cells," *Frontiers in Physiology* 9 (2018): 725.

356 Brandon J. Shad et al., "Daily Myofibrillar Protein Synthesis Rates in Response to Low – and High-Frequency Resistance Exercise Training in Healthy, Young Men," *International Journal of Sport Nutrition and Exercise Metabolism* 31, no. 3 (February 17, 2021): 209–16.

Another study had subjects train for 8 weeks and divided them into one group who trained once per day (performing 8 sets per exercise). One group trained twice per day (performing 4 sets per exercise, once in the morning and once in the evening). At the end of the study, the gains in muscle were the same between training twice per day and training once per day.[357] Another study compared once-a-day training to twice-a-day training and found similar gains in strength.[358] It should be mentioned that the strength gains were slightly better for twice a day training, so splitting your workouts into two sessions is an option if you are focused purely on strength. In a study in male weightlifters, athletes who trained twice a day had greater isometric strength, muscle activation, testosterone, and testosterone: cortisol ratio than those who did once-daily training. Despite these positive changes, muscle growth was the same, but favored the group that trained once a day (+3.2%) versus twice-a-day training (+2.1%).[359]

SUMMARY: There does not appear to be any advantage of training multiple times per day compared to a single session for muscle growth. If you love being in the gym and want to train twice a day, that's fine, but it does not appear to serve any extra muscle growth stimulus when training once per day when total exercise volume is similar. Multiple training sessions per day seem to elicit more favorable strength changes.

---

357 Daniel A. Corrêa et al., ~Twice-Daily Sessions Result in a Greater Muscle Strength and a Similar Muscle Hypertrophy Compared to Once-Daily Session in Resistance-Trained Men,~ *The Journal of Sports Medicine and Physical Fitness*, February 26, 2021.

358 Kai Shiau, Te Hung Tsao, and Chang Bin Yang, "Effects of Single Versus Multiple Bouts of Resistance Training on Maximal Strength and Anaerobic Performance," *Journal of Human Kinetics* 62 (June 2018): 231–40.

359 Michael Hartman et al., "Comparisons Between Twice-Daily and Once-Daily Training Sessions in Male Weight Lifters," *International Journal of Sports Physiology and Performance* 2 (July 1, 2007): 159–69.

CHAPTER SUMMARY

- Trained athletes have less of an increase in protein synthesis after exercise than untrained athletes and less damage.

- If they have recuperated properly, trained athletes can likely train a muscle group after 48 hours because protein synthesis has returned to baseline levels. This is dependent on their recovery capacity.

- Training a muscle group twice a week is superior to training a muscle group once a week.

- Training six days a week results in no greater strength and muscle growth than 3 days a week.

- Training twice a day does not increase muscle growth when the volume is similar between groups.

- Twice a day seems to favor better strength gains.

- Training volume seems to be the driving force behind increased muscle mass with increasing frequency.

CHAPTER 11:

SORE MUSCLES

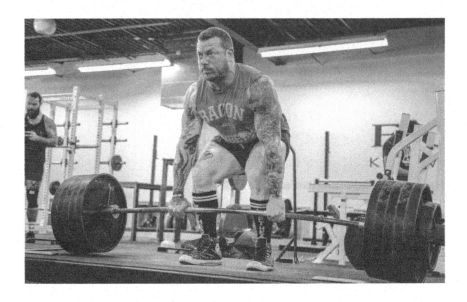

The most common method that people use to gauge if they had a good workout is sore muscles the next day. Your muscles ache, so that means you caused muscle damage and more muscle damage means more muscle growth...right? Muscle damage as a contributing factor to muscle growth has been a topic of discussion lately. Some scientists are changing their minds about how important muscle damage is for muscle growth.

MUSCLEGATE: SORE MUSCLES ARE A SIGN OF MUSCLE GROWTH.

THE TRUTH EXPOSED: Muscle soreness often occurs after intense exercise, and this is the gauge that lifters use to measure their previous workout. "NO PAIN, NO GAIN" is a common thought that you did not push yourself hard enough unless you were sore after your workout. Muscle damage leads to a cascade of events after exercise, leading to increased inflammation, cell swelling, and tenderness in the exercised area. These chemicals make nerve ending more sensitive, creating the perception of soreness. First, muscle soreness is a poor indicator of actual muscle damage.[360] When researchers compared how sore they felt after intense eccentric exercise, there was very little relationship between blood markers of muscle damage and subjects rating of soreness. In another study, scientists hooked up electrodes and electrically stimulated subjects' legs to maximally contract or had them perform exercise leg extension as hard as they could. Both groups experienced intense soreness after exercise. However, when looking at tissue samples of the muscle after exercise, the electrically stimulated muscle had much greater muscle damage than the exercise group, despite both groups feeling similar levels of muscle soreness. [361] This suggests that muscle soreness is not a good indicator of how much muscle damage has occurred. There is a large variability in how sore people are after exercise. Don't gauge soreness as a marker of how great your workout was or how much muscle damage you think occurred. In a study of college

---

360 Kazunori Nosaka, Mike Newton, and Paul Sacco, "Delayed-Onset Muscle Soreness Does Not Reflect the Magnitude of Eccentric Exercise-Induced Muscle Damage: DOMS and Muscle Damage," *Scandinavian Journal of Medicine & Science in Sports* 12, no. 6 (December 2002): 337–46.

361 R. M. Crameri et al., "Myofibre Damage in Human Skeletal Muscle: Effects of Electrical Stimulation versus Voluntary Contraction," *The Journal of Physiology* 583, no. Pt 1 (August 15, 2007): 365–80.

football players, athletes that reported feeling "better" driven by perceived levels of increased muscle soreness had a greater risk of injury.[362]

Research suggests that muscle soreness is not a good indicator of muscle growth. Studies have found that trained subjects experience muscle growth without muscle soreness.[363] One study tracked muscle growth over 10 weeks. The subjects experienced intense muscle soreness after the initial workout at 48 hours. In weeks 3 and 10, muscle soreness was very low after workouts. The subjects had an average ~14% increase in muscle growth at the end of the study. *Muscle growth had no relationship with any marker of muscle damage, such as soreness or blood markers of muscle damage (i.e., Creatine kinase).*[364] Other studies have found no difference in muscle size in those who reported high and low soreness.[365] A better indicator of muscle damage is strength loss. Of all the markers of muscle damage that are used (muscle soreness, swelling, range of motion, creatine kinase, etc.), muscle function related to force production is the most reliable indicator of muscle damage.[366]

After repeated bouts of resistance exercise, muscles become more resilient to muscle damage, and the body produces adaptive effects to protect against further muscle damage. This process is called the *repeated bout effect.* This means that with each workout, there is subsequently less damage occurring. The other concept to keep in mind is that long-distance

---

362 John A Sampson et al., "Subjective Wellness, Acute: Chronic Workloads, and Injury Risk in College Football," *Journal of Strength and Conditioning Research* 33, no. 12 (December 1, 2019): 3367–73.

363 Kyle L. Flann et al., "Muscle Damage and Muscle Remodeling: No Pain, No Gain?," *Journal of Experimental Biology* 214, no. 4 (February 15, 2011): 674–79.

364 Felipe Damas et al., "Resistance Training-Induced Changes in Integrated Myofibrillar Protein Synthesis Are Related to Hypertrophy Only after Attenuation of Muscle Damage," *The Journal of Physiology* 594, no. 18 (September 15, 2016): 5209–22.

365 Gederson K. Gomes et al., "High-Frequency Resistance Training Is Not More Effective Than Low-Frequency Resistance Training in Increasing Muscle Mass and Strength in Well-Trained Men," *Journal of Strength and Conditioning Research* 33 Suppl 1 (July 2019): S130–39.

366 Gøran Paulsen et al., ~Leucocytes, Cytokines and Satellite Cells: What Role Do They Play in Muscle Damage and Regeneration Following Eccentric Exercise?,~ 2012, 56.

running can cause lots of muscle damage and soreness and very little muscle growth. Most lifters don't feel like they exercised hard enough unless they can't move the next day. It is okay to be a little sore after exercise; that is normal, but those that seek more damage than is necessary for muscle growth can lead to a path of overtraining. Research has also shown that blood flow restriction training increases muscle growth without significant damage, suggesting that muscle growth is separate from muscle damage.[367] It has also been demonstrated that when subjects performed concentric only exercise (i.e., no eccentric contractions performed), there was a significant increase in lean mass, muscle thickness, and flexed arm circumference. Still, no evidence of training-induced muscle damage was observed.[368]

There is debate whether muscle damage is the true cause of muscle growth. This truly is a controversial subject and completely changes the way researchers look at muscle growth. For decades, it was believed that tension overload caused damage to the muscle, followed by protein synthesis and muscle growth. It should be stated that excess muscle damage will cause a loss of muscle size. In a 2001 study, researchers applied compression damage in which a weighted device was dropped from a fixed height on the rat's leg. Excess muscle damage resulted in a loss of muscle size and impaired regeneration. This again points to excess damage not being the driving force for muscle growth.[369] Therefore, there must be tension overload with damage for muscle growth to occur. In mice, excess downhill

367 J. P. Loenneke, R. S. Thiebaud, and T. Abe, "Does Blood Flow Restriction Result in Skeletal Muscle Damage? A Critical Review of Available Evidence," *Scandinavian Journal of Medicine & Science in Sports* 24, no. 6 (December 2014): e415-422.

368 Matt S. Stock et al., "The Time Course of Short-Term Hypertrophy in the Absence of Eccentric Muscle Damage," *European Journal of Applied Physiology* 117, no. 5 (May 1, 2017): 989–1004.

369 V. B. Minamoto, S. R. Bunho, and T. F. Salvini, "Regenerated Rat Skeletal Muscle after Periodic Contusions," *Brazilian Journal of Medical and Biological Research = Revista Brasileira De Pesquisas Medicas E Biologicas* 34, no. 11 (November 2001): 1447–52.

running causes excess muscle damage and inhibits muscle growth.[370] This suggests excess damage is not conducive for muscle growth.

Comparing blood flow restriction training to heavy resistance exercise further complicates the role of muscle damage and muscle growth. Both groups increased muscle mass, with the advantage towards heavy resistance exercise. The BFR group increased muscle mass without muscle damage or cell swelling. The heavy resistance exercise group had muscle damage in the first 3 weeks but was attenuated by week 6.[371] This again suggests that muscle damage should not be used to gauge muscle growth. If muscle damage were the predominant cause of muscle growth, one would expect muscle damage to occur after extended eccentric exercise. This does not occur due to the repeated bout effect, and muscles become more resilient to muscle damage. One study compared muscle damage response to concentric only vs. eccentric only lifting for ten weeks. In the eccentric-only training group, markers of muscle damage were elevated to a greater degree than in the concentric-only group at the beginning of the study. The subjects all experienced muscle soreness, as most people do after performing heavy eccentric exercises. Here is the shocker! By week 10, *markers of muscle damage were similar in both groups*, and neither group showed any indication of post-workout muscle damage.[372] This suggests that the muscle becomes more resistant to damage over time. Hence, the muscles learn to protect themselves from further damage.

Don't train for damage. Train enough to create an optimal stimulus, not excess muscle damage. I prefer a happy medium in which it's normal to

370 Alisson L. da Rocha et al., "Downhill Running Excessive Training Inhibits Hypertrophy in Mice Skeletal Muscles with Different Fiber Type Composition," *Journal of Cellular Physiology* 231, no. 5 (May 2016): 1045–56.

371 Fabiano Freitas Shiromaru et al., "Differential Muscle Hypertrophy and Edema Responses between High-Load and Low-Load Exercise with Blood Flow Restriction," *Scandinavian Journal of Medicine & Science in Sports* 29, no. 11 (November 2019): 1713–26.

372 Nikos V. Margaritelis et al., "Eccentric Exercise per Se Does Not Affect Muscle Damage Biomarkers: Early and Late Phase Adaptations," *European Journal of Applied Physiology* 121, no. 2 (February 2021): 549–59.

feel a little sore after a workout, but not to where you feel like your muscles have been obliterated. If you have no soreness, then maybe your intensity is too low, or your volume is too low. Just because you are not sore, don't assume you didn't have a good workout. The body has an amazing ability to become resilient to muscle damage. Muscle soreness should not be the sole indicator of basing your workout but a marker of a stimulus that has occurred, which should be used with other training variables such as muscle pumps, strength increases, fatigue, etc.

MUSCLEGATE: ECCENTRIC EXERCISES ARE MORE IMPORTANT FOR MUSCLE GROWTH

THE TRUTH EXPOSED: My first introduction to eccentric contractions was from fitness magazines. The article talked about how "eccentric contractions" were the most important part of the lift. The article described several studies in which eccentric only exercises resulted in muscle growth. I took away that concentric contractions were not that important, but both are equally important. You can lower the weight with more weight than you can lift. Your eccentric strength (i.e., lowering the weight) is about 20–40% greater than your concentric strength (lifting the weight), so naturally, this results in a greater amount of tension overload for the eccentric portion. I have seen many training partners that will use the leg press, and once the lifter pushes the weight forward, the spotter will push down on the weight, adding tension. Another common method is to use the leg extension or leg curl and lift with both legs and lower with one leg.

In studies that compare eccentric exercise to concentric exercise, there is greater muscle growth from eccentric exercise (10%) than concentric exercise (6.8%) due to a greater tension placed on the muscle through an eccentric contraction.[373] Remember, you can handle a greater weight lowering the weight than lifting. There is also evidence of greater type II muscle fiber growth during eccentric overloading exercise. One of the most impressive studies comparing traditional exercise to eccentric overload was a study performed on hockey players, which found that eccentric overload resulted in an 8.9% increase in quad muscle growth. In contrast, the traditional resistance exercise group gained 2.1%.[374] The problem with these studies is that most of the studies were performed on equipment not found in conventional gyms; as a result, we often create our own methods of eccentric overload, but it's very difficult to replicate an accentuated eccentric overload machine. The most common method is lifting with two arms and lowering with one arm (i.e., pulling down with a v bar handle with both hands and slowly lowering the weight with one arm). The same concept can be used with the legs, where you lift the weight with both legs and lower with one leg.

One study used a special squat machine that allowed a normal concentric contraction and an overloaded eccentric component (18–25%) compared to regular resistance exercise. The way this machine works is that you would lift with a weight of 300 pounds; the machine would lower with 375 lbs. At the end of the study, the group using the eccentric overload gained more strength in the first four weeks but failed to increase strength during the second four weeks. However, muscle growth gains were similar between the two groups.[375] The concentric/eccentric overload group had greater strength gains; however, muscle growth increased the same in both groups, despite the concentric/eccentric overload group using a 40%

---

373 Brad J. Schoenfeld et al., "Hypertrophic Effects of Concentric vs. Eccentric Muscle Actions: A Systematic Review and Meta-Analysis," *Journal of Strength and Conditioning Research* 31, no. 9 (September 2017): 2599–2608.

374 Oscar Horwath et al., "Isokinetic Resistance Training Combined with Eccentric Overload Improves Athletic Performance and Induces Muscle Hypertrophy in Young Ice Hockey Players," *Journal of Science and Medicine in Sport* 22, no. 7 (July 2019): 821–26.

375 Jamie Douglas et al., "Effects of Accentuated Eccentric Loading on Muscle Properties, Strength, Power, and Speed in Resistance-Trained Rugby Players," *Journal of Strength and Conditioning Research* 32, no. 10 (October 2018): 2750–61.

greater workload on the eccentric component.[376] It could be suspected that once tension overload reaches a certain threshold, no further increases in tension will stimulate muscle growth. Both groups were likely meeting their maximum threshold for tension, and further tension with the eccentric overload did not stimulate further muscle growth. Similar to once volume reaches a certain threshold, additional increases in sets result in no further increases in muscle growth.

Remember, in most studies comparing muscle growth responses to eccentric exercise directly to concentric exercise, the maximal eccentric exercise incorporated a heavier weight than the concentric portion. What if you equate the concentric and eccentric workloads, so they were equal? One study measured arm size and strength changes in response to groups that used a normal concentric contraction with an eccentric overload compared to a traditional resistance exercise program. Because eccentric overload uses a heavier weight, the researchers had the subjects in the traditional exercise group do an additional set to create an even total workload. The regular training groups did 4 sets of 75% of a 1 RM with concentric and eccentric contractions. The eccentric overload group did 3 sets of 75% a concentric 1RM and eccentric contractions with 120% of 1RM. To everyone's surprise, there was no difference in muscle growth even though both groups increased muscle strength at the end of the study.[377] The author suggested that the lack of changes in muscle could have been because of the advanced training status of the subjects, or longer than 9 weeks of training could have resulted in changes in muscle size.

---

376 Simon Walker et al., "Greater Strength Gains after Training with Accentuated Eccentric than Traditional Isoinertial Loads in Already Strength-Trained Men," *Frontiers in Physiology* 7 (2016): 149.

377 Jason P. Brandenburg and David Docherty, "The Effects of Accentuated Eccentric Loading on Strength, Muscle Hypertrophy, and Neural Adaptations in Trained Individuals," *Journal of Strength and Conditioning Research* 16, no. 1 (February 2002): 25–32.

In some cases, an excess of eccentric overloading can cause a decrease in muscle mass early in the training stages. Researchers had subjects use 5 sets of eccentric exercises with 110% of their 1-RM. The researchers measured the biceps circumference with MRI imaging. After the intense eccentric exercise, the subjects experienced soreness and elevated markers of muscle damage. Still, the most shocking finding was that *arm volume or size decreased* on three separate occasions at weeks 2, 3, and 8 weeks after exercise. The authors suspected the loss of arm volume was due to intense damage caused by eccentric exercise.[378] This again points to extreme muscle damage that can result in impaired muscle gains, with muscle damage far exceeding the body's ability to recuperate and grow. Also, keep in mind that heavy eccentric exercise that causes muscle damage will reduce the muscle's ability to store glycogen.[379] Thus, athletes will have impaired recuperation following intense eccentric exercise.

MUSCLE DAMAGE

 MUSCLE DAMAGE IS SEPERATE FROM MUSCLE GROWTH

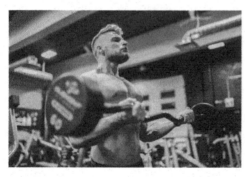

✓ MUSCLE DAMAGE IS A POOR INDICATOR OF MUSCLE GROWTH

✓ EXCESS MUSCLE DAMAGE CAN REDUCE MUSCLE GROWTH

✓ DON'T FOCUS ON MUSCLE DAMAGE

✓ NEW EXERCISES AND ECCENTRIC EXERCISE INCREASE MUSCLE DAMAGE

✓ MUSCLE DAMAGE BECOMES LESS OVER TIME (REPEATED BOUT EFFECT)

---

378 Jeanne M. Foley et al., "MR Measurements of Muscle Damage and Adaptation after Eccentric Exercise," *Journal of Applied Physiology* 87, no. 6 (December 1, 1999): 2311–18.

379 D. L. Costill et al., "Impaired Muscle Glycogen Resynthesis after Eccentric Exercise," *Journal of Applied Physiology (Bethesda, Md.: 1985)* 69, no. 1 (July 1990): 46–50.

CONCENTRIC AND ECCENTRIC EXERCISES RESULT IN DIFFERENT TYPES OF MUSCLE GROWTH

It's important to note that concentric and eccentric muscle contractions result in muscle growth, but it's achieved through contraction-specific modalities. The concentric portion or muscle shortening will increase muscle size diameter or cross-sectional area. Eccentric contractions stretch the muscle, which causes an increase in muscle growth by increasing fascicle length.[380] The easiest way to think about muscle fibers is thousands of thin wires bundles together; if you bend the wires (muscle contraction), the tension will be the greatest to the area directly applied (exercise angle), but you can also stretch those wires (eccentric contractions) by pulling at both ends apart. Studies have found that eccentric-only contractions cause muscle growth at the distal or furthest end of the muscle, whereas concentric contractions cause muscle growth in the middle region.[381] *This suggests that you need a combination of concentric and eccentric exercises for maximal muscle growth because each contraction causes different types of muscle growth.* As you will learn later, therefore, partials or half-reps' movements are sub-par for training adaptations because muscle stretch is important for muscle growth. Just keep in mind, always think how much damage you occur during exercise will determine when you can retrain that muscle, so if you are planning to add some eccentric overload partner-assisted contractions, plan for increased recovery time.

SUMMARY: Overloading the eccentric component results in more muscle damage and soreness at first. The muscle then protects itself from further damage through the repeated bout effect. After that, muscle damage and soreness are diminished. If you incorporate heavy eccentric exercise into

---

380 Martino V. Franchi, Neil D. Reeves, and Marco V. Narici, "Skeletal Muscle Remodeling in Response to Eccentric vs. Concentric Loading: Morphological, Molecular, and Metabolic Adaptations," *Frontiers in Physiology* 8 (July 4, 2017): 447.

381 M. V. Franchi et al., "Architectural, Functional and Molecular Responses to Concentric and Eccentric Loading in Human Skeletal Muscle," *Acta Physiologica (Oxford, England)* 210, no. 3 (March 2014): 642–54.

your routine, you will probably need to reduce your workout frequency to accommodate the excess muscle damage and soreness. If you are still sore, you should not work out again because you have not fully recovered.

CHAPTER SUMMARY

- Muscle soreness is not a good indicator of muscle growth.

- Muscle growth had no relationship with any marker of muscle damage, such as soreness or blood markers of muscle damage (i.e., creatine kinase).

- Different muscle groups recuperate from exercise at different rates depending on the tension exposure.

- More muscle damage does not mean more muscle growth.

- Muscle damage becomes less over time due to the repeated bout effect, but muscle growth still occurs.

- Excess muscle damage can reduce muscle growth.

- When using the same amount of weight, concentric contractions (lifting the weight) are highly fatiguing, whereas eccentric contractions (lowering the weight) are relatively fatigue-resistant.

CHAPTER 12:
PROGRAM JUMPING

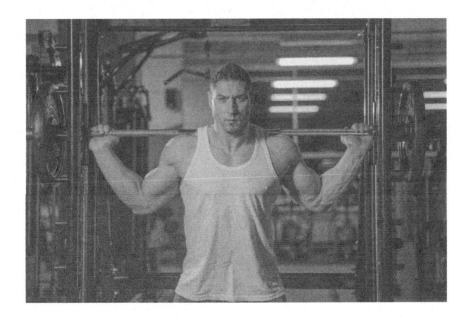

It is common for lifters who are frustrated with their lack of progress to use different training techniques and exercises. They will try advanced training techniques for a few weeks, such as supersets, dropsets, and rest-pause; after that, they will try something completely new. This is referred to as "program jumping." There is nothing wrong with program variety; however, there needs to be consistency in a workout routine. Constantly changing the workout exercise angle with different exercises may reduce your ability to adapt to a workout.

MUSCLEGATE: USE COMPLETELY DIFFERENT EXERCISES FOR MORE MUSCLE GROWTH

THE TRUTH EXPOSED: The research has consistently shown that changing exercises leads to higher motivation levels. It is tough to do the same exercises week after week without variety. One may question whether changing the sets, reps, duration of the contraction time, etc., on a weekly basis, can promote greater muscle growth?

Researchers measured quad growth in response to two different workout routines for 16 weeks. One leg did leg press and leg extension the same workout each time, and the other leg changed one variable each time to ensure that each workout was different; each group trained to failure. The variable group changed the exercise weight, volume, contraction type, and inter-set rest interval. Muscle protein synthesis was slightly higher for the varied group compared to the constant group. The total volume load (sets x reps x load) was higher in the varied group than in the constant group; however, leg growth was the same.[382] *Keep in mind they didn't change the exercise angle; they only changed a training variable* (i.e., load, volume, contraction type, and inter-set rest interval). This is consistent with various types of periodization programs that compare periodized to undulating programs in which, when the volume is similar, but the exercise intensity is changed; there are similar increases in muscle growth. Again, this points to a certain amount of training consistency with the same exercises, with the volume being the determining variable for muscle growth. There is nothing wrong with changing any of these variables; however, changing the exercise angle requires a new neurological adaptation to occur.

Some lifters like to change the exercise they do each time they exercise. A recent study compared training with just one exercise (i.e., the leg press on Monday, Wednesday, and Friday) to training each muscle group

---

382 Felipe Damas et al., "Myofibrillar Protein Synthesis and Muscle Hypertrophy Individualized Responses to Systematically Changing Resistance Training Variables in Trained Young Men," *Journal of Applied Physiology (Bethesda, Md.: 1985)* 127, no. 3 (September 1, 2019): 806–15.

3 times per week (leg press on Monday, half squat on Wednesday, hack squat on Friday). Total workout volume and intensity were matched in both groups. At the end of nine weeks, a combination of exercises resulted in a slight trend towards better overall muscle growth (12 different muscles sites) throughout the body. In contrast, the same exercise group failed to experience significant growth in 2 of the measured sites.[383] *Do not misinterpret the study; they performed the same exercises.* They did not use a new exercise each time they went to the gym. They just alternated leg exercises on Monday, Wednesday, and Friday. This study should not be misinterpreted to change your workout, so that every time you go to the gym, there is no consistency. It is perfectly fine to change exercises, but make sure it is consistent with a designated workout mesocycle.

The process of constantly changing the workout is commonly referred to as "muscle confusion" by bodybuilders. It advocates that frequently changing your workout will cause a greater increase in muscle growth. An example of muscle confusion would change the exercise every week. So, if you did the bench press last Monday, you should do incline dumbbells next Monday and decline bench the following Monday. In essence, you never do the same workout twice. In another study, subjects either performed a set workout routine in which they performed designated workout or a group in which they were allowed to randomly choose exercises from a workout app of over 80 different exercises. Their training volume was equated to be similar, and all sets were taken to failure. At the end of the study, the randomly chosen exercises found their workout more enjoyable, whereas the fixed routine resulted in decreased motivation. The 1-RM bench press went up about 4% in the fixed group and about .77% for the variation group. In terms of muscle growth, both groups similarly increased muscle growth, but *the group that performed the set workout routine had a slight advantage towards more muscle growth in parts of their legs (11%) as opposed to the*

---

383 Bruna Daniella de Vasconcelos Costa et al., "Does Performing Different Resistance Exercises for the Same Muscle Group Induce Non-Homogeneous Hypertrophy?," *International Journal of Sports Medicine* 42, no. 9 (July 2021): 803–11.

group that varied their workout each time (3%).[384] This study suggests that muscle confusion or changing your workout each time you go to the gym can lead to less strength and possibly muscle gains. Here is how muscle confusion can cause less muscle growth. The body adapts to training by protecting muscle from further damage after consistent training; if you constantly change the exercise each week, there is no adaptation because it is a new exercise, and there is constant muscle damage. One of the biggest mistakes lifters can make is going from one routine (i.e., drop-sets) to another (rest-pause) with no training consistency. Training variation is perfectly okay, but stick to consistent core lifts (i.e., multi-joint) for a training cycle and finish the workout with single-joint exercises at the end. For example, doing bench press and incline presses for six weeks, but each week performs a different type of cable crossover fly, dumbbell fly, or a pec deck. In sum, changing your workout too frequently can lead to impaired strength gains and muscle growth.

CHOOSE EXERCISE THAT DIRECTLY TARGETS MUSCLE GROUPS

If you need to improve your upper chest, doing more incline bench press makes sense than doing bench press and decline. Choose exercises that directly target the muscle groups you want to grow. Changing your workout can make it enjoyable and lead to a greater workout consistency rate; however, some evidence suggests that you may want to stick to a specific routine for a certain period has slight advantages. So, changing your workout will not make your muscles grow faster than doing the same routine. It is recommended that you keep certain core exercises constant throughout a training cycle, whereas isolation exercises can be varied frequently. This is consistent with a 2017 study in which subjects were assigned to

---

384 Eneko Baz-Valle et al., "The Effects of Exercise Variation in Muscle Thickness, Maximal Strength and Motivation in Resistance Trained Men," *PloS One* 14, no. 12 (2019): e0226989.

a fixed workout (had to perform the workout in a fixed order) or variability exercise group (self-selected the exercise for each muscle group). The group that had the freedom to choose the exercises they preferred for each muscle group had greater increases in upper body muscle mass.[385] The group that could choose their exercises still chose the same exercises in the majority of the 9 weeks (i.e., bench press, leg press, cable press down). This suggests there needs to be some consistency in workouts to gain muscle, and even when lifters are allowed to choose exercises, they stick to exercises that they enjoy doing. If you hate doing an exercise, or it causes joint discomfort, do not use it, and find an exercise that you enjoy and can do consistently. This is consistent with the above study; despite having a choice of a variety of different exercises, they used exercises they enjoyed performing a majority of their workouts.

MUSCLEGATE: ALL YOU NEED ARE THE BIG 3 EXERCISES FOR MAXIMAL MUSCLE GROWTH

THE TRUTH EXPOSED: The big three exercises commonly used for building mass are the squats, bench press, and deadlift. Other mass building exercises commonly used are the bent-over row, military presses, etc. Some may wonder if it is necessary to include accessory exercises (i.e., isolation exercises) with each body part. A common gym myth is that if you want to build mass, you need to do the bench, squat, and deadlift. Some have even said that you don't need other exercises, just these three lifts! Tension is applied to a different muscle region each time you change exercise angles. There are definite advantages to changing the exercise angles in your routine. Varying the exercise angles hits the muscle fibers from different areas, causing regional hypertrophy of that muscle. When you apply

---

385 Jacob T. Rauch et al., "Auto-Regulated Exercise Selection Training Regimen Produces Small Increases in Lean Body Mass and Maximal Strength Adaptations in Strength-Trained Individuals," *The Journal of Strength & Conditioning Research* 34, no. 4 (April 2020): 1133–40.

tension to a muscle, the whole muscle does not always grow uniformly. The muscle region most directly exposed to tension will grow, depending on the exercise variation. For example, the shoulder should be considered three different muscle groups: the front, side, and back. You need exercises that stimulate all three regions of the deltoids (i.e., military press, side lateral raises, rear deltoid raises). The quadriceps have four muscles (vastus lateralis, vastus medialis, rectus femoris, vastus intermedius). If you just perform squats, this will not maximize the growth of the quadriceps compared to a combination of different exercises. The classic study had one group train with smith machine squats while another group trained with machine squats, leg press, lunge, and deadlifts. The volume was the same for both groups, but the group that did a wide range of exercises resulted in a greater increase in muscle growth of the legs that trained the muscle from different angles compared to just squats.[386] Those that did a combination of squats, leg presses, deadlifts, and lunges led to greater increases in all four muscles of the quadriceps (vastus lateralis, vastus medialis, rectus femoris, vastus intermedius). In contrast, squats alone failed to increase in two muscle groups (rectus femoris and vastus medialis). A similar study had men train with leg extensions or squats for five weeks. The leg extensions increased muscle size in the area of the quadriceps called the rectus femoris, but the squat did not. The squat increased muscle size of the region of the leg called the vastus lateralis, but the leg extension did not.[387] This suggests you need a wide variety of exercises to stimulate multiple regions of a muscle for optimal muscle growth.

Others have found that a combination of exercises is needed to maximize hamstring growth. The hamstring muscles consist of the semitendinosus, semimembranosus, the biceps femoris. Nordic hamstring curls

386 Rodrigo M. Fonseca et al., "Changes in Exercises Are More Effective than in Loading Schemes to Improve Muscle Strength," *Journal of Strength and Conditioning Research* 28, no. 11 (November 2014): 3085–92.

387 Aitor Zabaleta-Korta et al., "The Role of Exercise Selection in Regional Muscle Hypertrophy: A Randomized Controlled Trial," *Journal of Sports Sciences* 0, no. 0 (July 10, 2021): 1–7.

display greater semitendinosus activity than biceps femoris activity.[388] Conversely, stiff-legged deadlifts present similar activity between the two muscles. This suggests that you need a wide variety of exercises to maximize hamstring muscle growth. Another misconception is that many lifters think the squat will increase hamstring muscle growth. Squats are great for quadriceps growth but result in little to no hamstring growth.[389] Therefore, you need seated hamstring curls, stiff-legged deadlifts, and glute-ham raises to maximize the growth of the hamstrings. Instead of the traditional "stick to the basics," if muscle growth is your goal, one should "hit muscles from a variety of angles."

Looking at how most people do calf raises, they often place the feet forward. One study had subjects train calf raises with their feet pointed in, pointed out, and forward. The group that pointed their toes out had better growth of the inner calf, the group that pointed their feet inward had more outer calf growth, and the group that pointed their feet forward had all the calf muscles grow equally.[390]

Similarly, the chest has an upper, middle, and lower region. It is three different muscles, so training with one particular exercise will not effectively stimulate all three muscles maximally. It was found that bench press alone led to the growth of the middle and lower region, while only the incline bench press led to a greater increase in the upper region of the chest.[391] In this study, researchers examined how different chest exercises

388 A. Hegyi et al., "Region-Dependent Hamstrings Activity in Nordic Hamstring Exercise and Stiff-Leg Deadlift Defined with High-Density Electromyography," *Scandinavian Journal of Medicine & Science in Sports* 28, no. 3 (March 2018): 992–1000.

389 Lawrence W. Weiss, Harvey D. Coney, and Frank C. Clark, "Gross Measures of Exercise-Induced Muscular Hypertrophy," *Journal of Orthopaedic & Sports Physical Therapy* 30, no. 3 (March 1, 2000): 143–48.

390 João Pedro Nunes et al., ~Different Foot Positioning During Calf Training to Induce Portion-Specific Gastrocnemius Muscle Hypertrophy,~ *The Journal of Strength & Conditioning Research* 34, no. 8 (August 2020): 2347–51.

391 SUENE F. N. CHAVES et al., "Effects of Horizontal and Incline Bench Press on Neuromuscular Adaptations in Untrained Young Men," *International Journal of Exercise Science* 13, no. 6 (August 1, 2020): 859–72.

influenced muscle growth. Subjects were randomly assigned to one of the three groups:

1. a horizontal bench press group

2. an incline bench press group

3. a combination (bench press + incline press) group.

The group that did the bench press first, followed by incline, did not increase the size of the upper region of the chest, compared to the group that did incline bench press first. This suggests that you should train the muscle groups you want to maximize *first!*

CHANGING BODY POSITIONS RESULTS IN DIFFERENT MUSCLE ACTIVATION

Changes in body positions can lead to increased muscle activation. For example, simply going from a seated dumbbell shoulder press to a standing dumbbell shoulder press leads to 8% greater front delt activation, 15% greater lateral delt activation, and 24% greater rear delt activation compared to the seated version.[392] Other examples of increasing activation of the lateral side of the deltoid would be to slightly lean into the position. For example, a leaning dumbbell side lateral raise in which you hang onto a post or gym apparatus with one hand and do a lateral extension with the other works the lateral head of the shoulder to a greater extent than a standing lateral raise.[393] Changing your stance from a narrow conventional-style deadlift (narrow stance) to a sumo style stance or using a trap

---

392 Atle H. Saeterbakken and Marius S. Fimland, "Effects of Body Position and Loading Modality on Muscle Activity and Strength in Shoulder Presses," *Journal of Strength and Conditioning Research* 27, no. 7 (July 2013): 1824–31.

393 P. J. McMahon et al., "Shoulder Muscle Forces and Tendon Excursions during Glenohumeral Abduction in the Scapular Plane," *Journal of Shoulder and Elbow Surgery* 4, no. 3 (June 1995): 199–208.

bar deadlift will increase quad activation. Whereas conventional deadlifts result in more activation of the lower back.[394]

Changing exercises and body positions are needed to maximize muscle growth; it is important to change exercises frequently, but not too often. There needs to be some consistency in your workouts. If you change your workout from day to day, this can be counterproductive.

CHAPTER SUMMARY

- Consistently using an exercise will result in better strength gains instead of frequently changing exercises.

- Changing an exercise routine too often may result in less favorable muscle growth.

- Changing the exercise angle can lead to increases in muscle growth of various muscle regions.

---

394 Rafael F. Escamilla et al., "An Electromyographic Analysis of Sumo and Conventional Style Deadlifts," *Medicine & Science in Sports & Exercise* 34, no. 4 (April 2002): 682–88.

CHAPTER 13:

METABOLIC TRAINING TO BUILD MUSCLE

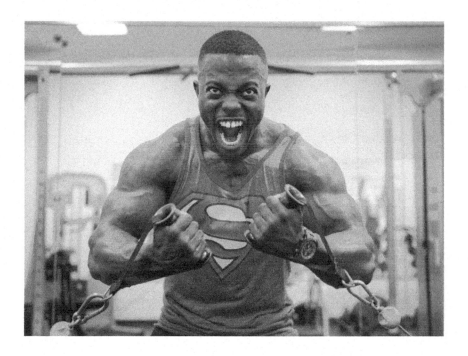

As mentioned previously, many lifters will use various techniques to increase exercise intensity and metabolic stress in a workout to increase muscle growth. Many of these techniques are popularized in fitness magazines such as *SuperSets*, *DropSets*, *Forced Reps*, *Pre-Exhaustion Training*, and *Rest-Pause* training. These techniques combine increasing metabolic stress and reducing rest periods in a workout. These training principles involve using a greater density of training in a shorter time.

MUSCLEGATE: SUPERSETS BUILD MUSCLE FASTER THAN TRADITIONAL EXERCISES

THE TRUTH EXPOSED: Supersets are a widespread technique in which you exercise two muscles (i.e., agonist and antagonist muscles) without rest between sets. The rationale is that, as one muscle gets fatigued, the opposite muscle can be exercised immediately after. A superset involves alternating exercises with opposed muscle groups to increase training volume and reduce total session time. For example, Supersetting arms involve exercising the biceps, followed immediately by the triceps. The advantage of Supersets is that it allows the antagonistic muscle to be exercised (e.g., triceps), which allows for the agonist muscle group (e.g., biceps) to rest. This allows for almost complete rest of an opposing muscle group, unlike a protocol integrating similar muscles. An example would be a set of biceps curls and then immediately performing a triceps extension. Another example would be performing leg extensions immediately followed by leg curls. Supersets allow you to perform more volume in a short time frame than traditional training.[395] Supersetting the bench press immediately followed by lat-pulldown and then resting for 180 seconds before the next superset resulted in 10% more weight lifted than traditional training, with 90 seconds of rest between each set.[396]

Supersets are most often seen with arm exercises. Researchers set out to determine if Supersets would result in bigger arms, but the caveat was that they used untrained subjects. One group of subjects did three sets of supersets (bicep curls followed immediately by triceps extensions). In contrast, the other group did traditional arms curls and triceps extensions—subjects trained to complete muscular failure on each set. At the end of the study,

---

395 Gabriel A. Paz et al., "Volume Load and Neuromuscular Fatigue During an Acute Bout of Agonist-Antagonist Paired-Set vs. Traditional-Set Training," *Journal of Strength and Conditioning Research* 31, no. 10 (October 2017): 2777–84.

396 Daniel W. Robbins, Warren B. Young, and David G. Behm, "The Effect of an Upper-Body Agonist-Antagonist Resistance Training Protocol on Volume Load and Efficiency," *Journal of Strength and Conditioning Research* 24, no. 10 (October 2010): 2632–40.

guess what? There were no differences in arm size between the groups, but the traditional group tended to have greater muscle growth.[397] It should be mentioned that the Superset group finished their work out faster than the traditional training group. As mentioned previously, when sets are taken to failure with a sufficiently heavy weight, muscle growth is virtually identical when comparing different techniques. Supersets can stimulate muscle growth in a shorter time because you can pack more tension on a muscle in a shorter time, but they are more fatiguing. Of all the advanced training techniques, supersets are the one lifting technique that can *increase performance* and volume. Ideally, using this approach, 2-minute rest between sets for compound movement would be a better option, whereas smaller muscle groups like the arms can be done without rest periods between sets. Supersets are highly fatiguing but are a great choice, for example, if you must get a workout done in 45 minutes. For example, subjects completed three resistance training protocols (Traditional exercise, Supersets, and Trisets), each with six exercises for 3 sets x 10 repetitions at 65% of a 3RM. During the traditional training protocol, all sets of one exercise were completed before moving on to the next exercise. In contrast, the Supersets (i.e., two consecutive exercises) and Trisets (three consecutive exercises) protocols were completed consecutively in one set before rest. The average session duration was greatest for the traditional training (42.3-min), compared to the Supersets (24.0-min) and Trisets training (17.7-min). Exertion levels were lower after the traditional training than after the Supersets and Trisets training. Session efficiency was much greater for Trisets training than for Supersets and Traditional training. However, Traditional training led to a restoration of muscle explosive power 24 hours post-training, yet this same measure was still reduced following Supersets and Trisets training. In sum, Supersets or Trisets training methods may allow for a sufficient amount of work to be completed in a short time frame. However, greater recuperation

397 Julius Fink et al., "Physiological Responses to Agonist–Antagonist Superset Resistance Training," *Journal of Science in Sport and Exercise*, October 18, 2020.

time is needed following both Supersets and Trisets training to minimize the effects of fatigue.[398]

EXAMPLE OF A SUPERSET:

- Leg Extension followed by Leg Curls
- Bicep Curls followed by Triceps Extensions
- Bench Press followed by Bent Over Rows

COMPOUND SETS

Another variation of the SuperSet is what's called *Compound Sets,* in which you can train two exercises *for the same muscle group without rest.* For example, a compound set is doing a lat pulldown immediately, followed by a bent-over row. Many people may wonder which is more effective. When performing supersets, is it better to use opposing muscle groups or similar muscle groups? One study compared compound sets using similar muscle groups (i.e., Five sets of leg press and knee extensions with no rest between sets). The Superset group used different muscle groups (bench press and knee extensions first, followed by Supersetting leg press and pec deck). The groups performed a similar work volume for both groups. At the end of the study, the compound group (using similar muscle groups) resulted in higher muscle activation and more muscle damage than using different muscle groups.[399] Another study compared the performance (maintaining velocity, power, and force) between compound sets with similar muscle groups compared (i.e., dumbbell bench, dumbbell press, and bench press) to using opposite muscle groups (i.e., bent over row and bench press). The

---

398 Jonathon J. S. Weakley et al., "The Effects of Traditional, Superset, and Tri-Set Resistance Training Structures on Perceived Intensity and Physiological Responses," *European Journal of Applied Physiology* 117, no. 9 (2017): 1877–89.

399 Michel A. Brentano et al., "Muscle Damage and Muscle Activity Induced by Strength Training Super-Sets in Physically Active Men," *Journal of Strength and Conditioning Research* 31, no. 7 (July 2017): 1847–58.

group that performed the opposing muscle groups maintained greater performance over the four sets than those that worked similar muscle groups without rest.[400]

Another study compared compound sets with different rest period durations. Sixty resistance-trained men were divided into two groups, one who trained chest muscles and the other trained back muscles. Both chest and back groups performed three exercises: Chest: barbell bench press, incline barbell bench press, and a chest butterfly; Back: lat pull-down, back row, and shoulder extension. Both groups completed 3 sets x 8 reps per exercise at 80% of their 1RM. Each group completed three trials requiring the participants to rest for 60-, 90-, and 120-sec between sets and exercises. The researchers found that a greater number of repetitions were performed in the 120-second rest periods between sets compared to the 90 – and 60-second conditions, and a greater number in the 90-second condition, compared to the 60-second condition. Since volume is a key driver of muscle growth, it may be wise to take a minimum of 120 seconds' rest between sets for muscle growth. For both the chest and back groups, the training volume of the second exercise was substantially reduced by shorter rest periods (60 – and 90-sec) compared to the first exercises.[401] This suggests that using shorter rest intervals results in greater metabolic stress and elicits a reduction in training volume.

Since compound sets cause more damage, does it result in more muscle growth? Researchers compared compound sets to a traditional weight training routine for 12 weeks. The compound set group performed Smith machine squats and leg press with no rest between exercises. In contrast, the conventional training group alternated between Smith machine

---

400 Jonathon J. S. Weakley et al., "The Effects of Superset Configuration on Kinetic, Kinematic, and Perceived Exertion in the Barbell Bench Press," *Journal of Strength and Conditioning Research* 34, no. 1 (January 2020): 65–72.

401 Filipe Matos et al., "Effect of Rest Interval Between Sets in the Muscle Function During a Sequence of Strength Training Exercises for the Upper Body," *Journal of Strength and Conditioning Research* 35, no. 6 (June 1, 2021): 1628–35.

squat and leg press sets, with one-minute rest between sets. The total work-out volume is equal in both groups. The strength gains and muscle growth were identical at the end of the study.[402] The key point is that volume is the most important factor for muscle growth, but compound and supersets allow for greater density in a shorter time frame.

Superset sets (opposing muscle groups) may be a better choice than compound sets (similar muscle groups) when you are short on time. Furthermore, Supersets results in less performance decline and also less muscle damage. If you are looking for an occasional day in which you want to shock muscles with an intense workout, use compound sets occasion-ally. If you are looking for the optimal amount of time to rest between sets (1, 2, 3 minutes or rest until you feel ready with no time constraint), 2.5 minutes seemed to be the optimal time to rest between sets without adversely affecting volume and performance when using antagonist mus-cle groups.[403]

COMPOUND SETS EXAMPLE:

- **Bench Press followed by Pec Deck Flyes**
- **Bent Over Rows followed by Lat Pulldowns**

SUMMARY: If you are crunched on time and need to get a quick work-out, supersets with opposing muscle groups seem to result in the optimal workout with less performance decline than compound sets with similar muscle groups. It should also be pointed out that compound sets with two similar muscle groups (incline and bench press) resulted in lower training

---

402 Justin J. Merrigan, Margaret T. Jones, and Jason B. White, "A Comparison of Compound Set and Traditional Set Resistance Training in Women: Changes in Muscle Strength, Endurance, Quantity, and Architecture," *Journal of Science in Sport and Exercise* 1, no. 3 (November 1, 2019): 264–72.

403 Cristiano Behenck et al., "The Effect of Different Rest Intervals Between Agonist-Antagonist Paired Sets on Training Performance and Efficiency," *Journal of Strength and Conditioning Research*, June 9, 2020.

volume. This was more likely due to the greater muscle fatigue caused by training two muscle groups with no rest between sets.

DROP SETS

A *Drop Set* consists of using a weight and completing the set until failure, then without rest, as the name implies, lowering or dropping the weight and doing additional sets to failure. This is done several times, depending on how many drop sets you want to perform. There are many names that drop sets have been referred to as running the rack, strip sets, etc. Drop sets normally decrease the weight by 20–25% with each drop set and are taken to complete failure. An example of a drop set would be doing leg extensions with 100 pounds until muscular failure, immediately dropping the weight to 90 pounds and completing an exercise to muscular failure, and then without rest, dropping the weight to 80 pounds until muscular failure. The principle of drop sets allows for more volume in a shorter period. The fitness magazines like to use sexy headlines like "Shock Your Muscles into Growth with Drop-Sets!"

MUSCLEGATE: DROP SETS BUILD MUSCLE FASTER THAN TRADITIONAL EXERCISES

THE TRUTH EXPOSED: Most of the studies that have compared drop sets to traditional resistance exercises have found similar muscle growth when the total workout volume is similar.[404,405] There is one study that favored muscle growth when using drop sets over traditional resistance

---

404 Vitor Angleri, Carlos Ugrinowitsch, and Cleiton Augusto Libardi, "Crescent Pyramid and Drop-Set Systems Do Not Promote Greater Strength Gains, Muscle Hypertrophy, and Changes on Muscle Architecture Compared with Traditional Resistance Training in Well-Trained Men," *European Journal of Applied Physiology* 117, no. 2 (February 2017): 359–69.

405 Hayao Ozaki et al., "Effects of Drop Sets with Resistance Training on Increases in Muscle CSA, Strength, and Endurance: A Pilot Study," *Journal of Sports Sciences* 36, no. 6 (March 2018): 691–96.

exercise when the volume was equated.[406] It may be worth considering adding a dropset after your normal sets. One study found that including a single drop set resulted in greater muscle mass than a traditional weight training routine.[407] The addition of the single drop set resulted in a 23% greater volume than the conventional weight training group. This suggests that it was not the drop set itself that increased muscle growth, but the extra volume of performing an additional set. Drop sets should be used for machine-based exercises and limited for high coordination exercises such as the squat and bench press due to high fatigue and greater risk of form deterioration.

DOES THE AMOUNT OF WEIGHT DROPPED EACH SET DETERMINE MUSCLE GROWTH?

A drop set is normally performed without a rest period, but does the amount of weight dropped each set affect muscle growth? Researchers compared lifters who trained biceps to failure for three sets and another group that trained to failure the first set but reduced the weight by 5 or 10% on the following sets. At the end of the study, all the groups had a similar increase in muscle growth. Still, the group that dropped their weight by 10% found it was less stressful.[408] This suggests that when you are training to failure with arms, you can drop the weight by either 5 or 10 pounds, and it won't make a difference for muscle growth if you are training to failure.

406 Fink, J., Schoenfeld, B.J., Sakamaki-Sunaga, M. et al. Physiological Responses to Agonist–Antagonist Superset Resistance Training. J. of SCI. IN SPORT AND EXERCISE 3, 355–363 (2021).

407 Kazushige Goto et al., "Muscular Adaptations to Combinations of High – and Low-Intensity Resistance Exercises," *Journal of Strength and Conditioning Research* 18, no. 4 (November 2004): 730–37.

408 Bruce M. Lima et al., "Planned Load Reduction Versus Fixed Load: A Strategy to Reduce the Perception of Effort With Similar Improvements in Hypertrophy and Strength," *International Journal of Sports Physiology and Performance* 13, no. 9 (October 1, 2018): 1164–68.

Another study set out to determine what training principle is the king of muscle growth. Researchers compared pyramid sets (gradually increasing the weight of each set), drop-sets, and traditional resistance exercises for 12 weeks. The training volume was similar for all the training groups. They also used fairly heavy training percentages in their first set (65–85%) and used a high exertion level. At the end of the study, all groups had similar increases in muscle growth; interestingly, the drop-sets and pyramid sets trained to muscular failure, whereas the traditional exercise did not, but all groups had similar increases in muscle growth.[409] *It also highlights that training volume appears to be the most important determining factor for muscle growth rather than the routine or metabolic stress.*

In a 2021 study, drop-sets were found to result in certain regions of muscle growth that were not found with traditional training. The resistance training study lasted eight weeks, with the drop set protocol consisting of a 5RM load to failure, reducing the load by 20% to failure again, then reducing the load by 10-15% to failure. The traditional strength protocol consisted of 15RM to failure. At the end of eight weeks, although both had similar increases in leg muscle mass, however, drop-sets resulted in a superior increase in the rectus femoris (front middle region of the thigh).[410] Upon analysis of the training volume, the drop set group resulted in a higher training volume. The greater exercise volume with dropsets was suggested to enhance hypertrophy of the targeted rectus femoris compared to the traditional strength training group.

Drop-sets can be a great way to add volume to single-joint exercises such as bicep curls, triceps extensions, and calf training to bring up lagging body parts. Drop sets incorporate many stimulating reps in a very short

409 Alysson Enes et al., "Rest-Pause and Drop-Set Training Elicit Similar Strength and Hypertrophy Adaptations Compared to Traditional Sets in Resistance-Trained Males," *Applied Physiology, Nutrition, and Metabolism,* July 14, 2021.

410 Dorian Varović et al., "Drop-Set Training Elicits Differential Increases in Non-Uniform Hypertrophy of the Quadriceps in Leg Extension Exercise," *Sports (Basel, Switzerland)* 9, no. 9 (August 29, 2021): 119.

time. Drop sets are great for a time-efficient workout. It would be extremely fatiguing to use drop sets for multi-joint exercises such as the squat, bench press, and other major body parts. The risk to reward ratio is too high for using drop-sets with squats because of fatigue's rapid deterioration with exercise form. It's best to use drop sets for single – joint exercises where you can easily drop the weight yet maintain proper form.

AN EXAMPLE FOR CABLE ARM WORKOUT DROP SET

100 lbs. x 10 reps or till failure, immediately drop the weight

90 lbs. x till failure, immediately drop the weight

80 lbs. x till failure, immediately drop the weight

70 lbs. x or till failure, immediately drop the weight

MUSCLEGATE: REST–PAUSE BUILDS MUSCLE FASTER

THE TRUTH EXPOSED: When the concept of rest-pause was introduced; it made complete sense to build muscle based on the practical application of combining high tension and metabolic stress caused by short rest periods. Rest-pause training involves performing a set until failure, resting for 10–30 seconds, and repeating this method for how many times you desire. The beauty of rest-pause is that it allows lots of fatigue in a short amount of time, resulting in a greater increase in training volume. Another benefit with rest-pause is that you are not decreasing the weight like drop-sets, so tension is constant. Rest-pause is similar to drop-sets, but you use the same weight throughout the entire sets instead of dropping the weight and taking brief rest periods between sets. The advantage of rest-pause is that many stimulating reps are being performed in a brief period. Several studies have found that rest-pause training resulted in greater gains in lean muscle mass than traditional training.[411] Another advantage of rest-pause is that it requires less time to complete. For example, one study found that traditional exercise took 57 minutes to complete and 35 minutes for rest-pause training. After six weeks, strength gains were similar between groups, but the rest-pause group achieved greater muscle growth in the legs (11%) vs. traditional training (1%).[412] It should be mentioned that a major limitation of the study comparing the groups was that traditional training completed 3 sets of 6 reps with 80% of a 1-RM and were not taken to failure. In contrast, the rest-pause group trained their first set to complete muscular failure. Another study found that rest-pause resulted in a 32.6% greater increase in volume and 26.8% greater repetitions performed than traditional training—rest-pause training results in greater muscle activation and no greater post-workout fatigue than conventional exercise.[413] A 2021 meta-analysis of cluster sets, rest-pause, and other studies involving shortened rest periods found that rest-pause was equally effective as traditional resistance exercise, with less fatigue development.[414]

A 2019 study found that rest-pause training resulted in greater muscle growth in only the thighs than a traditional resistance exercise group.[415] This led to a flurry of training articles in the fitness magazines to *Get Bigger in Less Time with Rest-Pause Training*. Keep in mind that the study did a

---

411 Jonathan M. Oliver et al., "Greater Gains in Strength and Power with Intraset Rest Intervals in Hypertrophic Training," *Journal of Strength and Conditioning Research* 27, no. 11 (November 2013): 3116–31.

412 Jonato Prestes, Ramires A. Tibana, et al., "Strength and Muscular Adaptations After 6 Weeks of Rest-Pause vs. Traditional Multiple-Sets Resistance Training in Trained Subjects," *The Journal of Strength & Conditioning Research* 33 (July 2019): S113.

413 Paul W. M. Marshall et al., "Acute Neuromuscular and Fatigue Responses to the Rest-Pause Method," *Journal of Science and Medicine in Sport* 15, no. 2 (March 2012): 153–58.

414 Timothy B. Davies et al., "Chronic Effects of Altering Resistance Training Set Configurations Using Cluster Sets: A Systematic Review and Meta-Analysis," *Sports Medicine (Auckland, N.Z.)* 51, no. 4 (April 2021): 707–36.

415 Jonato Prestes, Ramires A Tibana, et al., "Strength and Muscular Adaptations After 6 Weeks of Rest-Pause vs. Traditional Multiple-Sets Resistance Training in Trained Subjects," *Journal of Strength and Conditioning Research* 33 Suppl 1 (July 2019): S113–21.

complete body workout, but only the thighs resulted in greater gains in muscle mass.

A 2021 study shook up the research community when a study titled "Rest-pause and drop-set training elicit similar strength and hypertrophy adaptations compared to traditional sets in resistance-trained males" was released. They took resistance-trained men and assigned them to a rest-pause, drop-set, or a traditional weight training group. This study only consisted of leg exercises comprised of squats, leg press, and leg extensions. The total workout volume was similar for all the groups. At the end of the study, the rest-pause group resulted in the greatest increase in squat strength. *All the groups had similar increases in muscle mass.* Another study compared pyramid sets (gradually increasing the weight of each set), drop-sets, and traditional resistance exercises for twelve weeks. The training volume was similar for all the training groups. They also used fairly heavy training percentages in their first set (65–85%) and used a high exertion level. At the end of the study, all groups had similar increases in muscle growth; interestingly, the drop-sets and pyramid sets trained to muscular failure, whereas the traditional exercise did not and still had similar increases in muscle growth.[416] This study suggests that volume is the biggest driver of muscle growth, rather than any particular training principle. If you want to incorporate any of these techniques into your training routine, it may be worth experimenting with, but they don't seem to be superior to regular resistance exercise.

If you compare advanced training techniques with similar volumes such as pre-exhaustion training, forced reps, supersets, and traditional resistance exercise, all result in altered metabolic stress (lactate), muscle activation, and muscle swelling. However, there are no differences in

416 Enes, A., Alves, R. C., Schoenfeld, B. J., Oneda, G., Perin, S. C., Trindade, T. B., Prestes, J., & Souza-Junior, T. P. (2021). Rest-pause and drop-set training elicit similar strength and hypertrophy adaptations compared with traditional sets in resistance-trained males. Applied physiology, nutrition, and metabolism = Physiologie appliquee, nutrition et metabolisme, 46(11), 1417–1424.

muscle growth compared to traditional resistance exercise when training volume is similar.[417] Rest-pause may be advantageous to use during a high-volume phase. Rest-pause resulted in a significantly greater number of effective reps and the total number of reps completed, indicating that total training volume was significantly greater (approximately 1.6 x greater) without decreasing acute repetition performance than traditional resistance exercise.[418]

REST-PAUSE CALF WORKOUT EXAMPLE

Pick a weight to perform 10–15 reps until failure.

Rest for 15–30 seconds.

Perform another set to failure in the same manner.

Rest another 15–30 seconds.

Perform another set to failure in the same manner.

MUSCLEGATE: PRE-EXHAUSTION TRAINING INCREASES MUSCLE GROWTH FASTER

THE TRUTH EXPOSED: The theory behind pre-exhaustion training is that if you perform an isolation exercise before a multi-joint exercise; the muscle is pre-fatigued, which results in greater muscle fiber activation during the compound joint exercise. The classic example is leg extensions performed by squats or leg press. Pre-exhaustion training has been advocated to "bring up weak body parts." The premise of pre-exhaust training is based on maximally fatiguing the muscle. The truth is, just the opposite occurs. When researchers measured muscle activation, pre-exhaustion

---

417 William Wallace et al., "Repeated Bouts of Advanced Strength Training Techniques: Effects on Volume Load, Metabolic Responses, and Muscle Activation in Trained Individuals," *Sports (Basel, Switzerland)* 7, no. 1 (January 6, 2019): E14.

418 James J. Tufano et al., "Cluster Sets vs. Traditional Sets: Levelling out the Playing Field Using a Power-Based Threshold," *PLOS ONE* 13, no. 11 (November 26, 2018): e0208035.

training with leg extensions before the leg press *resulted in a decrease in muscle activation* of the quadriceps.[419] Compared to traditional resistance exercises, subjects performed fewer reps in the leg press after pre-exhaustion training. A 2007 study investigated smaller muscle groups being performed before larger muscle groups. On one visit, they performed free-weight bench press, seated machine shoulder press, seated machine triceps extension, leg press, leg extension, and leg curl. On the second visit, they performed the exercises in reverse order. *When single-joint exercises precede, multi-joint exercises resulted in a decrease in the total number of repetitions.* This suggests that multi-joint exercises should be performed first for muscle growth.[420] Similar results have been found for the upper body. When pec deck flies were performed before bench press exercise; peck deck exercise performed immediately before bench press exercise led to similar muscle activation of the anterior deltoid and pectoralis major muscles; however, they observed the increase in triceps activation and the worst performance during the bench press exercise with pre-exhaustion.[421] The study suggests that performing pre-exhaustion exercise is no more effective in increasing the activation of the pre-fatigued muscles than during multi-joint exercises. Furthermore, to maximize the performance in a specific resistance exercise, this exercise should be placed at the beginning of the training session.

The final nail in the coffin for pre-exhaustion training was a 2019 study in which subjects performed either 3 sets of leg presses to failure or did one set of leg extensions until failure and immediately performed leg press to failure for nine weeks. *At the end of the study, muscle growth*

419 Jesper Augustsson et al., "Effect of Pre-Exhaustion Exercise on Lower-Extremity Muscle Activation during a Leg Press Exercise," *Journal of Strength and Conditioning Research* 17, no. 2 (May 2003): 411–16.

420 Walace Monteiro, Roberto Simão, and Paulo Farinatti, ~Manipulation of Exercise Order and Its Influence on the Number of Repetitions and Effort Subjective Perception in Trained Women,~ *Revista Brasileira de Medicina Do Esporte* 11 (March 1, 2005).

421 Gentil, P., Oliveira, E., de Araújo Rocha Júnior, V., do Carmo, J., & Bottaro, M. (2007). Effects of exercise order on upper-body muscle activation and exercise performance. Journal of strength and conditioning research, 21(4), 1082~1086.

responses were the same between both groups.[422] Others have reported similar findings that pre-exhaustion results in no greater muscle growth than traditional training.[423] It should come as no surprise since both groups trained to failure. These results suggest that pre-exhaustion will not lead to greater muscle growth.

PRE-EXHAUSTION EXAMPLE:

Leg Extension followed immediately by squats.

Chest flyes followed immediately by bench press

SUMMARY: All these intensity techniques promote better muscle pumps and increase the density of a training protocol in a short time. If you are looking for a deep dive into all the research on these training principles, I would recommend the review article, "No Time to Lift? Designing Time-Efficient Training Programs for Strength and Hypertrophy: A Narrative Review." The authors concluded that advanced training techniques, such as supersets, drop sets, and rest-pause training, roughly halves training time compared to traditional training while maintaining training volume. However, these methods are probably better at inducing hypertrophy than muscular strength, and more research is needed on longitudinal training effects.[424] You will undoubtedly get a great pump with any of these techniques. Still, when the volume is similar, these exercise principles result in similar muscle growth to traditional resistance exercise. If you are going to use these techniques, use them sporadically, as they can increase fatigue.

---

422 Trindade TB, Prestes J, Neto LO, et al. Effects of Pre-exhaustion Versus Traditional Resistance Training on Training Volume, Maximal Strength, and Quadriceps Hypertrophy. Front Physiol. 2019;10:1424.

423 James Peter Fisher et al., "The Effects of Pre-Exhaustion, Exercise Order, and Rest Intervals in a Full-Body Resistance Training Intervention," *Applied Physiology, Nutrition, and Metabolisme = Physiologie Appliquee, Nutrition Et Metabolisme* 39, no. 11 (November 2014): 1265–70.

424 Iversen, V. M., Norum, M., Schoenfeld, B. J., & Fimland, M. S. (2021). No Time to Lift? Designing Time-Efficient Training Programs for Strength and Hypertrophy: A Narrative Review. Sports medicine (Auckland, N.Z.), 51(10), 2079–2095.

These techniques help get in and out of the gym *faster* by increasing the workout volume, but the research does not suggest that they are *superior* to traditional training when volume is similar. Another training technique to boost volume is to have a good training partner that motivates you during exercise. When lifters were tested on the bench press with and without a training partner, on average, when they had a spotter, they performed almost 2 more reps per set and with less exertion.[425] This was just one session; imagine taking these results and spreading them over a year of training.

These techniques will work better for smaller muscle groups, such as the calves, arms, etc. When you train smaller body parts, greater peripheral fatigue (muscles) is tolerated. These techniques are great to use if you need to get in and out of the gym faster, but continued use can lead to greater training stress, excess fatigue, and longer recuperation times. In a review titled *Maximizing Muscle Hypertrophy: A Systematic Review of Advanced Resistance Training Techniques and Methods,* the author made the following key points about these advanced techniques:[426]

- Athletes may consider advanced training techniques to provide an additional stimulus to break through plateaus, prevent monotony, and reduce the time of training sessions.

- To maintain high time efficiency of training, the use of agonist/ antagonist supersets, drop sets, and cluster sets may provide an advantage to the traditional approach.

---

425 Andrew Sheridan et al., "Presence of Spotters Improves Bench Press Performance: A Deception Study," *Journal of Strength and Conditioning Research* 33, no. 7 (July 2019): 1755–61.

426 Michal Krzysztofik et al., "Maximizing Muscle Hypertrophy: A Systematic Review of Advanced Resistance Training Techniques and Methods," *International Journal of Environmental Research and Public Health* 16, no. 24 (December 4, 2019): E4897.

CHAPTER SUMMARY:

- Supersets (two back-to-back exercises using opposing muscle groups) can stimulate muscle growth in a shorter time because you can pack more tension on a muscle in a shorter time. However, they are not superior to traditional training when the volume is similar.

- Compound Sets (using similar muscle groups) result in higher muscle activation and more muscle damage than supersets.

- Compound sets result in similar muscle gains to traditional exercise.

- Supersets allow for greater performance than Compound Sets.

- Drop-sets involve dropping the weight each set but result in similar muscle growth as traditional exercise when volume is similar.

- Cluster sets, rest-pause, and other studies involving shortened rest periods found that rest-pause was equally effective as traditional resistance exercise with less fatigue development.

- Pre-exhaustion training leads to decreased performance and does not lead to greater increases in muscle growth.

CHAPTER 14:

RANGE OF MOTION

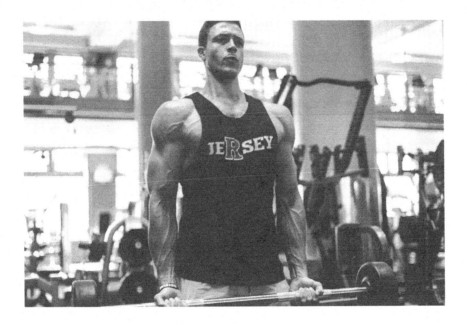

Range of motion is the degree to which a muscle is actively stretched during a repetition. It has been traditionally recommended that you perform a full range of motion with each repetition, so the muscle is fully contracted, followed by lowering the weight, so the muscle is fully stretched. A partial range of motion or half movement means that the movement does not fully stretch the muscle. If you think about the tension placed on a muscle, it sets x reps x weight and *distance*. The most obvious example that is seen is the leg press. Lifters will load up the leg press until it is full of 45's, lower the weight a few inches, and lift it to a full position. They may use a heavier weight, but the total tension placed on the muscle is reduced because the distance the weight has traveled is exponentially smaller than doing a full range of motion. Remember that tension and stretch are both equally important for muscle growth. When using a partial rep, you can handle more weight, so more weight results in greater muscle tension, which means greater muscle growth…right?

MUSCLEGATE: PARTIALS ARE BETTER FOR MUSCLE GROWTH

THE TRUTH EXPOSED: It's been suggested that using partial reps allows more weight, increasing muscle growth; the greater tension causes a compression-like effect on the muscle, creating metabolic stress. When you perform a full range of motion, different muscle fibers are activated by stretch. Although most people perform partial reps using a much heavier weight, researchers wanted to see the effects of a full range of motion vs. a partial range of motion using a similar weight. Researchers had subjects complete either triceps extension with either a full or a partial range of motion. The weights were progressively increased over eight weeks. The researchers measured metabolic stress, strength, muscle activation, and muscle growth. At the end of the study, partial reps resulted in greater metabolic stress, muscle activation, and muscle size in the triceps than a full range of motion.[427] Another study found that biceps muscle growth was similar between full (9.7%) and partial reps (7.8%), despite the full range of motion groups using 36% lower training volume.[428] Hold on! Before you start using partial reps for every exercise, these were just two studies. These were both single-joint exercises (triceps extensions and bicep curls). What about multi-joint exercises, such as the squat or bench press? A full range of motion resulted in greater increases in muscle mass than partial

427 Masahiro Goto et al., "Partial Range of Motion Exercise Is Effective for Facilitating Muscle Hypertrophy and Function Through Sustained Intramuscular Hypoxia in Young Trained Men," *The Journal of Strength & Conditioning Research* 33, no. 5 (May 2019): 1286–94.
428 Ronei S. Pinto et al., "Effect of Range of Motion on Muscle Strength and Thickness," *Journal of Strength and Conditioning Research* 26, no. 8 (August 2012): 2140–45.

movements for the legs.[429,430] A 2020 meta-analysis found a full range of motion resulted in more growth in four studies (three lower body and one upper body), growth was similar between the partial and a full range of motion in one lower body study and one upper body study found more growth with partial reps.[431] Thus, all lower-body results favor a full range of motion for muscle growth. If you think about a partial squat, the bottom part of the squat is completely neglected, which results in less stretch on the muscles. Stretching a muscle with a full range of motion is necessary for muscle growth.

A 2021 meta-analysis examining 16 published studies reported that a full range of motion results in more muscle growth and strength improvement in the legs than a partial range of motion.[432] One study found that when examining muscle growth responses in the leg extension, performing partials with the muscle stretched in the bottom portion of the leg extension, a full range of motion, and a full range of motion and partials combined resulted in similar muscle growth responses in the legs. *The key takeaway from this study is that muscles stretched at long muscle lengths, despite being a partial rep, can cause similar hypertrophy to a full range of motion training.*[433] Does this mean you should use partial ranges of motion for all exercises? Remember, this is just one study, but it sug-

---

429 Gerard E. McMahon et al., "Impact of Range of Motion during Ecologically Valid Resistance Training Protocols on Muscle Size, Subcutaneous Fat, and Strength," *Journal of Strength and Conditioning Research* 28, no. 1 (January 2014): 245–55.

430 K. Bloomquist et al., "Effect of Range of Motion in Heavy Load Squatting on Muscle and Tendon Adaptations," *European Journal of Applied Physiology* 113, no. 8 (August 2013): 2133–42.

431 Brad J Schoenfeld and Jozo Grgic, "Effects of Range of Motion on Muscle Development during Resistance Training Interventions: A Systematic Review," *SAGE Open Medicine* 8 (January 1, 2020): 2050312120901559.

432 Jesús G. Pallarés et al., ~Effects of Range of Motion on Resistance Training Adaptations: A Systematic Review and Meta-Analysis,~ *Scandinavian Journal of Medicine & Science in Sports* 31, no. 10 (2021): 1866–81.

433 Pedrosa, G. F., Lima, F. V., Schoenfeld, B. J., Lacerda, L. T., Simões, M. G., Pereira, M. R., Diniz, R., & Chagas, M. H. (2021). Partial range of motion training elicits favorable improvements in muscular adaptations when carried out at long muscle lengths. European journal of sport science, 1–11. Advance online publication.

gests that stretching a muscle is extremely important for muscle growth, even if it is not being taken through a full range of motion. The study also suggests that doing partials with a stretched muscle, for example, when doing leg curls having the hamstrings fully stretched at the beginning of the movement and then using a partial rep, can be effective as a full range of motion. Again, this was just one study, but the initial results are exciting, suggesting that partial reps with a stretched muscle can be effective as a full range of motion.

Here is an example of doing an exercise with a partial rep with stretched muscle length.

- Doing a lat pull down with the lats stretched and doing a partial range of movement.

- Doing a bicep curl would be to stretch the bicep off a preacher curl, lift it halfway up, and stretch the muscle again.

- Doing a dumbbell fly with the pecs stretched and doing a partial rep.

You want to stretch the muscle as far as possible; stretching the muscle can increase anabolic signaling pathways independent of tension.[434] Certain animal studies have shown that just by stretching a muscle with tension, you can increase muscle growth. The greater stretch of the hamstrings induced by seated leg curls results in more hamstrings growth than lying leg curls.[435] This same concept can explain why deep squats grow the glutes

---

434 David W. Russ, "Active and Passive Tension Interact to Promote Akt Signaling with Muscle Contraction," *Medicine and Science in Sports and Exercise* 40, no. 1 (January 2008): 88–95.

435 Sumiaki Maeo et al., "Greater Hamstrings Muscle Hypertrophy but Similar Damage Protection after Training at Long versus Short Muscle Lengths," *Medicine and Science in Sports and Exercise* 53, no. 4 (April 1, 2021): 825–37.

more than shallow squats because deep squats stretch the glutes more.[436] A recent 2021 study found that stretching the hamstrings before and during rest periods between squats led to increases in hamstring growth. The non-stretching group showed no increases in hamstring growth.[437]

The further the resistance or weight is away from a joint, the greater the tension your muscles will need to generate to overcome the resistance and weight lifted (longer muscles have a reduced ability to generate force). Keep in mind that the *combination of tension and stretching a muscle optimizes muscle growth*. For example, when you do a partial rep for a leg press, you start with the legs fully extended; not performing a full eccentric repetition is where all the muscle growth happens. Doing a partial rep without a fully stretched muscle is not conducive for muscle growth. The current research indicates that passive, low-intensity stretch does not result in beneficial changes in muscle growth. However, the research suggests that intense stretch training may stimulate muscle growth, particularly with weights or added between active muscle contractions.[438] This suggests that a combination of tension and muscle stretch is necessary for muscle growth. A meta-analysis of 26 studies found that isometric contractions in the stretched position increased muscle growth more than in a contracted position.[439] You may want to consider holding the muscle in a stretched position and contracting the muscle. For example, doing a leg curl and contracting the muscle while in the stretched position.

---

436 Keitaro Kubo, Toshihiro Ikebukuro, and Hideaki Yata, "Effects of Squat Training with Different Depths on Lower Limb Muscle Volumes," *European Journal of Applied Physiology* 119, no. 9 (September 2019): 1933–42.

437 Thiago Barbosa Trindade et al., "Pre-Stretching of the Hamstrings Before Squatting Acutely Increases Biceps Femoris Thickness Without Impairing Exercise Performance," *Frontiers in Physiology* 11 (2020): 769.

438 João Pedro Nunes et al., ~Does Stretch Training Induce Muscle Hypertrophy in Humans? A Review of the Literature,~ *Clinical Physiology and Functional Imaging* 40, no. 3 (May 2020): 148–56.

439 Dustin J. Oranchuk et al., "Isometric Training and Long-Term Adaptations: Effects of Muscle Length, Intensity, and Intent: A Systematic Review," *Scandinavian Journal of Medicine & Science in Sports* 29, no. 4 (April 2019): 484–503.

Stretching alone will not have a very big impact on muscle growth; otherwise, we would see jacked yoga instructors everywhere. For example, one study had subjects complete a static stretching program for six weeks with calf stretches. The groups stretched their calves once per week or three times per week. At the end of the study, neither muscle strength nor muscle size was changed regardless of the stretching frequency.[440] It's the combination of tension and stretch that increases muscle growth. If you experiment with partial reps, include them in workouts that use a full range of motion. A 2004 study found that a combination of full and partial squats resulted in a greater squat increase than just using a full range of motion.[441] As noted above, partial reps with the muscle in a stretched position was just as effective as doing a full repetition. Experiment with doing a few sets of a full range of motion, and your last set, when you are fatigued, use one set of partial reps. It may cause more muscle growth.

Keep in mind that you should not be performing an excessive range of motion by performing an exercise. Your range of motion should be done safely and feels comfortable to you. If, while doing the movement, you feel an excessive strain on your joints, then reduce the range of motion to where it becomes comfortable. The excellent news for people who don't like to stretch is that resistance training is comparable to passive stretching for increasing joint range of motion.[442]

---

440 Shigeru Sato et al., "The Effects of Static Stretching Programs on Muscle Strength and Muscle Architecture of the Medial Gastrocnemius," *PLOS ONE* 15, no. 7 (July 9, 2020): e0235679.

441 Caleb D. Bazyler et al., "The Efficacy of Incorporating Partial Squats in Maximal Strength Training," *Journal of Strength and Conditioning Research* 28, no. 11 (November 2014): 3024–32.

442 José Afonso et al., ~Strength Training versus Stretching for Improving Range of Motion: A Systematic Review and Meta-Analysis,~ *Healthcare* 9, no. 4 (April 2021): 427.

MUSCLEGATE: YOU SHOULD NEVER STRETCH BECAUSE IT REDUCES MUSCLE GROWTH

THE TRUTH EXPOSED: For years it was suggested that static stretching could reduce muscle soreness. However, a review of the literature concluded that stretching does not reduce soreness, regardless of whether the stretching is performed before or after the training bout.[443] There has been an anti-stretching campaign because a few studies have shown that stretching before exercise can reduce performance. It has been found that static stretching before exercise can reduce strength, reduce repetitions completed, and even reduce muscle growth compared to those that do not stretch before exercise.[444] The rubber band analogy is the most common way of thinking about how stretching too long can affect your power production. If you stretch a rubber band and let it go, it recoils, but if you stretch that rubber band back for an extended period, it loses its recoil ability and will not fly forward as far. The same principle applies to stretching for prolonged periods of time before exercise. Two factors determine whether stretching before a workout can decrease performance: duration and the intensity of the stretch.

Studies suggest if you hold a static stretch for less than a minute, it's not detrimental to performance.[445] *60 seconds is the max upper limit.* I would probably recommend less (<10 seconds). If you are going to stretch, do not perform prolonged static stretching, which is the traditional sitting on the ground. Stretch the muscle for 30 seconds or more, and then directly work out. How many times have you stretched and then immedi-

---

443 Robert D. Herbert, Marcos de Noronha, and Steven J. Kamper, "Stretching to Prevent or Reduce Muscle Soreness after Exercise," *The Cochrane Database of Systematic Reviews*, no. 7 (July 6, 2011): CD004577.

444 Roberto Moriggi Junior et al., "Effect of the Flexibility Training Performed Immediately before Resistance Training on Muscle Hypertrophy, Maximum Strength and Flexibility," *European Journal of Applied Physiology* 117, no. 4 (April 2017): 767–74.

445 Anthony D. Kay and Anthony J. Blazevich, "Effect of Acute Static Stretch on Maximal Muscle Performance: A Systematic Review," *Medicine and Science in Sports and Exercise* 44, no. 1 (January 2012): 154–64.

ately performed a squat? The research may not apply to real-world lifting because most studies have subjects stretch and immediately perform an exercise. Other studies have shown that if you stretch and then wait ten minutes, there is an increase in performance.[446] Short duration stretching for 20 seconds had no impact on reducing performance.[447] Also, the studies that have found that stretching reduces performance have used static stretching to the point of pain (85% pain), whereas stretching with low-intensity stretches (50% pain) has shown no reductions in performance.[448] It may be better to stretch after your workout or stretch at night if you are worried about it. If the stretches are short and low intensity, there will be minimal effects on performance. Low-intensity stretching has been found to improve recovery, possibly by increasing blood flow to the muscle.[449] A recent study divided men into three groups: a.) Static stretching, b.) dynamic stretching, and c.) control group. The static stretching group performed 2 different stretches for 2 sets of 20 seconds (i.e., a total of 80 seconds of stretching). In contrast, the dynamic stretch group performed 15 repetitions by moving their limb continuously through a challenging range of motion. Both groups stretched to a mild discomfort level. At the end of the study, all groups reported similar increases in muscle growth and strength.[450] The key point is that the subjects did not overly stretch their muscles (i.e., <20 seconds each stretch), and they kept the discomfort

446 Evan Peck et al., "The Effects of Stretching on Performance," *Current Sports Medicine Reports* 13, no. 3 (June 2014): 179–85.

447 João B. Ferreira-Júnior et al., ~Effects of Static and Dynamic Stretching Performed Before Resistance Training on Muscle Adaptations in Untrained Men,~ *Journal of Strength and Conditioning Research*, September 17, 2019.

448 Paulo H. Marchetti et al., "Different Volumes and Intensities of Static Stretching Affect the Range of Motion and Muscle Force Output in Well-Trained Subjects," *Sports Biomechanics*, August 29, 2019, 1–10.

449 Nikos C. Apostolopoulos et al., "The Effects of Different Passive Static Stretching Intensities on Recovery from Unaccustomed Eccentric Exercise – a Randomized Controlled Trial," *Applied Physiology, Nutrition, and Metabolism = Physiologie Appliquee, Nutrition Et Metabolisme* 43, no. 8 (August 2018): 806–15.

450 João B. Ferreira-Júnior et al., ~Effects of Static and Dynamic Stretching Performed Before Resistance Training on Muscle Adaptations in Untrained Men,~ *Journal of Strength and Conditioning Research*, September 17, 2019.

level at a 5. The studies that have found stretching interfered with muscle growth stretched before exercise, with a pain value between 8 and 10 and stretched for 30 seconds.[451]

The best way to stretch is to perform either static or *dynamic warm-ups*, in which you "move while stretching." An example would be squatting up and down with no weight before squats getting a full range of motion, or a walking lunge would be another form of a dynamic warmup. It's also been found that dynamic stretching after static stretching can counteract the adverse effects of static stretching.[452]

STRETCHING BETWEEN SETS *MAY* INCREASE MUSCLE GROWTH

In the previous chapter, we learned that supersets (exercising a muscle group, then immediately exercising an opposing muscle) group are an effective way to increase exercise volume. Many people do a set and then rest sitting and doing nothing. Several studies have found that stretching the opposite muscle group you exercise can increase performance.[453,454] For example, stretching the back while doing chest, stretching the hamstrings while doing leg extensions. Two studies have shown that stretching between sets may be beneficial. In one study, subjects either rested between sets or stretched between sets. The stretching consisted of low intensity, low pain stretching between sets for 30 seconds. At the end of the study,

451 Roberto Moriggi Junior et al., "Effect of the Flexibility Training Performed Immediately before Resistance Training on Muscle Hypertrophy, Maximum Strength and Flexibility," *European Journal of Applied Physiology* 117, no. 4 (April 2017): 767–74.

452 Iain M. Fletcher and Bethan Jones, "The Effect of Different Warm-up Stretch Protocols on 20 Meter Sprint Performance in Trained Rugby Union Players," *Journal of Strength and Conditioning Research* 18, no. 4 (November 2004): 885–88.

453 Humberto Miranda et al., "Acute Effects of Antagonist Static Stretching in the Inter-Set Rest Period on Repetition Performance and Muscle Activation," *Research in Sports Medicine (Print)* 23, no. 1 (2015): 37–50.

454 G. Paz et al., "Strength Performance Parameters and Muscle Activation Adopting Two Antagonist Stretching Methods before and between Sets," *Science & Sports* 31, no. 6 (December 1, 2016): e173–80.

there was a trend for greater muscle growth for the legs, whereas the other body parts did not benefit.[455] The other study found that stretching the calves between sets leads to greater muscle growth.[456] Contrary to this, a study that had subjects stretch between sets found no difference in muscle growth in the chest.[457] There is no concrete proof that stretching between sets will increase muscle growth, but it certainly won't hurt as long as the stretches are low intensity and don't cause pain.

CHAPTER SUMMARY

- Partial reps seem to work best for the arms, not the legs.

- Most research supports using a full range of motion for muscle growth.

- A combination of full and partial range of motion can be used to get the benefits of both worlds.

- Stretching a muscle at full length is a potent stimulus of muscle growth.

- Keep stretching before exercise to less than 20-60 seconds.

- Do Not Stretch to the point of intense pain before exercise.

- Dynamic warmups such as arm swings, walking lunges, walking knee raises are effective ways to warm up.

- Stretching the muscle between sets may increase muscle growth, but more research is needed.

---

455 Alexandre L. Evangelista et al., "Interset Stretching vs. Traditional Strength Training: Effects on Muscle Strength and Size in Untrained Individuals," *Journal of Strength and Conditioning Research* 33 Suppl 1 (July 2019): S159–66.

456 Simpson et al., "Stretch Training Induces Unequal Adaptation in Muscle Fascicles and Thickness in Medial and Lateral Gastrocnemii." Scandinavian journal of medicine & science in sports, 27(12), 1597–1604.

457 Tanuj Wadhi et al., "Loaded Inter-Set Stretching for Muscular Adaptations in Trained Males: Is the Hype Real?," *International Journal of Sports Medicine*, August 10, 2021.

CHAPTER 15:

MIND MUSCLE CONNECTION

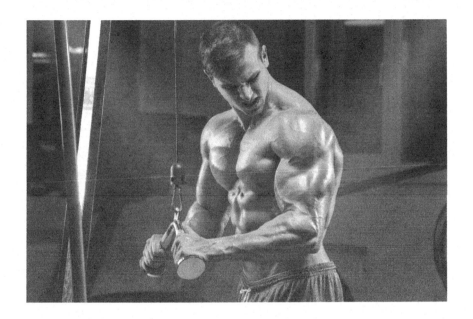

FOCUS ON THE MUSCLE

One of my favorite motivational speakers is *CT Fletcher*. CT Fletcher is a bodybuilder who underwent heart replacement surgery but still trains daily for those of you who do not know. Despite his doctors telling him to stop exercising, CT is still in the gym today. I would highly recommend his YouTube page for more motivating stories. In his older training videos before his heart surgery, CT had a famous saying; he would train his biceps and scream, *"I COMMAND YOU TO GROW!"* He would focus on squeezing the muscle as hard as possible for each rep. Other bodybuilders used to talk about focusing on the muscle each repetition and squeezing the muscle. If you watch the classic bodybuilding classic movie *Pumping Iron*,

Arnold Schwarzenegger said, *"Each rep, I focus on the muscle growing!"* Are you just lifting the weight each rep, or are you consciously focused on the muscle each rep and actively squeezing the muscle each repetition? Does the mind have any role in making your muscles grow each repetition?

MUSCLEGATE: JUST LIFT THE WEIGHT TO GET BIGGER

THE TRUTH EXPOSED: We realize that not all reps are created equal. There is a popular phenomenon called the *mind-muscle connection,* in which you actively focus on the muscle each repetition. It is not uncommon to see personal trainers touching a person's muscle while doing a set and telling them to squeeze the muscle. Is this all more bodybuilding voodoo science? Certainly not! Many lifters will get so focused on adding more weight and doing more reps that they forget that actively focusing on the muscle can increase muscle growth. If you are a powerlifter, then total weight lifted is your primary goal. Building muscle, not weight, is your primary goal if you are a bodybuilder.

Actively focusing on the muscle, each repetition results in more muscle fibers activated during a set. If you are a personal trainer, verbally telling your client to squeeze the muscle can be beneficial. Researchers had subjects train and were given verbal commands on the bench press such as "squeeze the muscle" for the pecs and triceps, or they were not told anything and allowed to just train. At lower intensities (50% of a 1RM), there was 22% greater pec muscles activation for those given verbal instructions to focus on the muscle. However, at a heavier weight (80% of a 1RM), there was less muscle activation (13%), despite being told to focus on the muscle.[458] At lower intensities (50% of a 1RM), triceps activity was 26% greater,

---

458 Benjamin J. Snyder and Wesley R. Fry, "Effect of Verbal Instruction on Muscle Activity during the Bench Press Exercise," *Journal of Strength and Conditioning Research* 26, no. 9 (September 2012): 2394–2400.

whereas there was no difference at 80%. This suggests that the mind-muscle connection may work well when training with lighter weight but not as effective with heavier weights. It also emphasizes the importance of giving verbal cues to your clients to contract the muscle with each repetition. The mind-muscle connection seems to work better for increasing muscle growth with single-joint exercises, such as the bicep curl or triceps extensions. If you are looking to build muscle, the mind-muscle connection of actively squeezing the muscle may be incorporated during light weight training periods. Still, it will not be effective with heavy weight training.

Another study investigated whether focusing on squeezing the muscle "thinking about it or internal cues" or having someone give you instructions "external cues" or "c'mon two more reps!!" Muscle activation was greater with internal cues of actively focusing on squeezing the muscle than those verbally told to squeeze the muscle.[459] This again points to actively squeezing the muscle for greater muscle activation and muscle growth. A follow-up study compared movement speed and mind-muscle connection. At *slow movement speeds* (50% of a 1-RM), subjects who were mentally focused on the muscle could increase muscle activation; however, at fast and explosive speeds, they could not increase muscle activation despite being told to mentally focus on the muscle.[460] This goes back to earlier concepts that the mind-muscle connection may work best with lighter weight; in contrast, it becomes less effective at heavier weights or if you are lifting the weight fast or explosively.

For bodybuilding, mentally focusing on squeezing the muscle may be better for muscle growth, since you are recruiting more muscle fibers. A study by muscle guru Brad Schoenfeld found that mentally focusing on

---

459 David C. Marchant and Matt Greig, "Attentional Focusing Instructions Influence Quadriceps Activity Characteristics but Not Force Production during Isokinetic Knee Extensions," *Human Movement Science* 52 (April 2017): 67–73.

460 Joaquin Calatayud et al., "Influence of Different Attentional Focus on EMG Amplitude and Contraction Duration during the Bench Press at Different Speeds," *Journal of Sports Sciences* 36, no. 10 (May 2018): 1162–66.

the contracting muscle *led to greater muscle growth of the biceps*, but for some reason, not the quads.[461] Subjects were instructed to mentally focus on squeezing the muscle or told verbally to "do another rep!" This may be because it is much easier to mentally focus on a single-joint exercise with smaller muscle groups like the bicep and triceps instead of training to large muscle groups like the quadriceps. Similar results were found with the lats. When subjects were instructed by a trainer to focus on a muscle group resulted in greater lat activation compared to just lifting the weight without focusing on the muscle.[462] Focusing on the muscle and squeezing the muscle each rep will decrease the number of repetitions, but do not let this bruise your ego. Just as the research above has described, there was greater muscle activation and greater muscle growth when lifters actively focused on squeezing the muscle. The advantage of using the mind-muscle connection is that it allows for a lighter weight but still enhances muscle growth. This can be an excellent tool for someone who needs to take a break from heavy lifting without sacrificing losing muscle. Using mind-muscle techniques can be especially beneficial during a deload when your purpose is recovery.

IS MUSCLE GROWTH ALL IN YOUR HEAD?

The mind is a powerful way to gain muscle. Many people classify themselves as 'hard-gainers,' but could this all be a mindset? If you believe you can't gain muscle, this could be a self-fulfilling prophecy. Researchers had participants receive genetic testing and perform exercise. One group of subjects was told they had "bad genes" for exercise performance. Even though some subjects had "good genes" that predisposed them to perform better

461 Brad Jon Schoenfeld et al., "Differential Effects of Attentional Focus Strategies during Long-Term Resistance Training," *European Journal of Sport Science* 18, no. 5 (June 2018): 705–12.

462 Benjamin J. Snyder and James R. Leech, "Voluntary Increase in Latissimus Dorsi Muscle Activity during the Lat Pull-down Following Expert Instruction," *Journal of Strength and Conditioning Research* 23, no. 8 (November 2009): 2204–9.

when they were told they had "bad genes" deceptively before their exercise bout, they performed worse. Simply thinking you have "bad genes" seemed to influence the outcome of the study results. This suggests that if you think you have "bad genes," it is a self-fulfilling outcome.[463] It could be the same reason why people who call themselves "Hardgainers" or "non-responders" never gain muscle because they believe they can't gain muscle.

The placebo effect is well documented in the fitness world. How many times have you bought a supplement and "felt" it was putting on muscle only to find out it was all in your head? The most striking example of this is a study in which subjects were told they were getting "steroids" in a weightlifting study. The "steroids" were nothing more than a placebo, but the lifters increased their total strength on the bench, squat, and deadlift by 100 pounds![464] There should be some positive expectations in your training that you will put on new muscle while you are training; if you think you will not gain muscle, then more than likely, you won't. In a study titled, "The top-down influence of ergogenic placebos on muscle work and fatigue," published in the *European Journal of Neuroscience*, researchers reported a 22% increase in strength in trained athletes who were told they were given high dose caffeine but received a placebo.[465] In another study, individuals were given a placebo comprising two milk-sugar tablets, 8–10 minutes before testing. They were told that the substance consisted of a "strong combination of amino acids and that the strength effects were immediate!" The placebo group increased strength in the bench press and seated leg press. In contrast, when the subjects were told they were given a placebo the previous experimental bout and re-tested, their strength declined to

---

463 Bradley P. Turnwald et al., "Learning One's Genetic Risk Changes Physiology Independent of Actual Genetic Risk," *Nature Human Behaviour* 3, no. 1 (January 2019): 48–56.

464 "Anabolic Steroids: The Physiological Effects of Placebos – This Study Is One of Three in an Investigation of the Short and Long Term Effects of an Anabolic Steroid (Dianabol) upon Human Performance – Ariel Dynamics,".

465 Antonella Pollo, Elisa Carlino, and Fabrizio Benedetti, "The Top-down Influence of Ergogenic Placebos on Muscle Work and Fatigue," *European Journal of Neuroscience* 28, no. 2 (2008): 379–88.

the same as the control group.[466] This suggests that if you believe something is working, it will! Scientists are just beginning to see how powerful the mind is for enhancing strength and possibly even muscle growth. A 2017 study found that when kickboxers utilized mental imagery in their routine resulted in greater strength increases. The group that performed mental imagery had increased testosterone and reduced cortisol and heart rate, resulting in lower training stress promoting a more favorable hormonal response to training.[467] This suggests the mind has a powerful outcome on eliciting favorable effects on performance and muscle growth.

CHAPTER SUMMARY

- Giving verbal cues to your clients if you are a personal trainer increases muscle activation.

- The mind-muscle connection works better with light weight and does not seem to be effective with heavier weights.

- Mental focusing on the muscle can increase muscle growth.

- The placebo effect has a powerful effect on performance.

---

466 Vasandreas Kalasountas, Justy Reed, and John Fitzpatrick, "The Effect of Placebo-Induced Changes in Expectancies on Maximal Force Production in College Students," *JOURNAL OF APPLIED SPORT PSYCHOLOGY* 19 (February 14, 2007): 116–24.

467 Maamer Slimani et al., "Effects of Mental Training on Muscular Force, Hormonal and Physiological Changes in Kickboxers," *The Journal of Sports Medicine and Physical Fitness* 57, no. 7–8 (August 2017): 1069–79.

CHAPTER 16:

EXERCISE ORDER

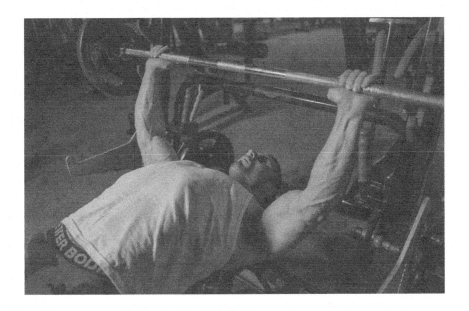

It is often recommended that you start with multi-joint exercises first, followed by single-joint exercises. A typical lifter would always train chest before triceps. It has been emphasized that all workouts should begin with multi-joint exercises first.

MUSCLEGATE: EXERCISE ORDER HAS NO IMPACT ON MUSCLE GROWTH

THE TRUTH EXPOSED: Most people in the gym will say they want to grow a specific body part more, but rarely change their workout order of exercises. For example, how often have you heard someone say that their calves won't grow, yet every time they train them, it's at the end of the workout! If you want to get a body part to grow, train it first. In the *Encyclopedia of Bodybuilding,* Arnold Schwarzenegger wrote he had weak calves for much of his career; he prioritized them by training them first every workout. It wasn't until he started training his calves first, did he truly grow his calves.

The exercise order should be based on what muscle you want to stimulate, independent of whether it's a multi-joint or a single-joint exercise. Remember, in the earlier chapter, that incline bench press performed before bench press resulted in greater muscle growth of the upper pecs. In contrast, incline performed after the bench press did not result in significant growth of the upper pecs. We have already discussed how pre-exhaustion training with a single-joint exercise (leg extension) followed by a multi-joint exercise (squat) results in similar muscle growth when the squat is performed first when both are taken to complete muscular failure. A meta-analysis of 11 studies found no impact of exercise order on muscle growth; however, for strength, whatever exercise you perform first had the greatest impact on strength gains.[468] The study found that exercise order had no effect on muscle groups such as the arms, deltoids, and quads, but it may adversely affect other muscle groups like the chest. A previous study in 2018 found that performing multi-joint exercises first had a small favorable effect on the legs. In contrast, other body parts, such as the arms, had

---

468 Nunes, J. P., Grgic, J., Cunha, P. M., Ribeiro, A. S., Schoenfeld, B. J., de Salles, B. F., & Cyrino, E. S. (2021). What influence does resistance exercise order have on muscular strength gains and muscle hypertrophy? A systematic review and meta-analysis. European journal of sport science, 21(2), 149–157.

no meaningful impact.[469] It should also be mentioned that a combination of machines and free weight exercises can be used for workout motivation and hitting muscle groups from a wide variety of exercise angles. For years, it was said that free weights are superior to machines for muscle growth, but a recent study in which subjects performed either free weights or machine exercises led to a similar increase in muscle growth.[470] In this study, men and women trained for eight weeks on different exercise modalities (i.e., free weight squat and smith machine leg press). The free-weight squat increased their 1RM free weight squat by 21.3%, whereas those using a Smith machine improved free-weight squat 1RM by 13.1%. Both groups had similar increases in lean muscle mass. Another 2021 meta-analysis of 16 studies found that training with free weights led to greater gains in strength in free weight exercises, whereas training with machines led to greater increases in machine weight strength.[471] The study reinforces the concept of training specificity, which means strength improvements are greater with whatever exercise you perform regularly (i.e., free weight or machines). A similar study compared the effects of training one multi-joint exercise (leg press) or two single-joint exercises (leg extension and kickback) on strength and the transferability of strength between exercises. The single-joint exercises group improved 6RM in leg extension and kickback more than the leg press, while the multi-joint exercise group improved leg press 6RM more than kickback.[472] This reinforces the concept that you get stronger in the exercises that you perform regularly. Also, the gains in lean

---

469 Avelar et al., "Effects of Order of Resistance Training Exercises on Muscle Hypertrophy in Young Adult Men."

470 Shane R. Schwanbeck et al., "Effects of Training With Free Weights Versus Machines on Muscle Mass, Strength, Free Testosterone, and Free Cortisol Levels," *Journal of Strength and Conditioning Research* 34, no. 7 (July 2020): 1851–59.

471 Kyle A. Heidel, Zachary J. Novak, and Scott J. Dankel, "Machines and Free Weight Exercises: A Systematic Review and Meta-Analysis Comparing Changes in Muscle Size, Strength, and Power," *The Journal of Sports Medicine and Physical Fitness*, October 5, 2021.

472 Nicolay Stien et al., "Training Specificity Performing Single-Joint vs. Multi-Joint Resistance Exercises among Physically Active Females: A Randomized Controlled Trial," *PLOS ONE* 15, no. 5 (May 29, 2020): e0233540.

mass were similar for both free weights and machines. Muscle growth is increased by muscle tension. Whether free weights or machines apply tension does not seem to make a difference. This is best supported by earlier studies in which cam or variable resistance exercise (i.e., Nautilus machines have been advocated to result in superior muscle growth because tension is applied over the entire range of motion) results in similar muscle growth as traditional machines.[473,474] As mentioned earlier, variable resistance push-up bands can produce similar increases in strength and size as traditional bench press exercises. These studies point to that despite different loading modalities, all can produce muscle hypertrophy as long as tension is applied for sufficient time.

The chest seems to be an important muscle group to train first. If you think about it, the deltoids, triceps, and biceps are still being used in the bench press and lat pull-downs, etc. The chest is not being exercised in other exercises. If you perform triceps exercises before incline or bench press, then more than likely, your performance will be negatively affected because your triceps have been pre-fatigued. However, your arms are still being exercised during chest movement, so the lower training reps won't likely affect muscle size because they have already had many stimulating reps from the bench press. If you want to grow your chest, it's best to start with chest exercises first. This is precisely what happened when researchers had subjects perform four weight training protocols:

- Barbell bench press plus lying barbell triceps press.

- Lying barbell triceps press plus barbell bench press.

- Barbell bench press.

---

473 Michał Staniszewski, Andrzej Mastalerz, and Czesław Urbanik, "Effect of a Strength or Hypertrophy Training Protocol, Each Performed Using Two Different Modes of Resistance, on Biomechanical, Biochemical and Anthropometric Parameters," *Biology of Sport* 37, no. 1 (March 2020): 85–91.

474 Simon Walker et al., "Variable Resistance Training Promotes Greater Fatigue Resistance but Not Hypertrophy versus Constant Resistance Training," *European Journal of Applied Physiology* 113, no. 9 (September 1, 2013): 2233–44.

- Lying barbell triceps press.

Interestingly, pec growth (5.6%) was lower in the group that performed lying triceps extensions before the bench press. Pec growth was greater following the bench press (9.1%) and bench press followed by lying triceps extensions had similar muscle growth (10.6%). Triceps growth was similar regardless of exercise order, whether they did the bench press first followed by triceps extensions or triceps extension first followed by bench press.[475] It could be body parts such as the arms are getting additional muscle activation with other exercises such as chest and back that exercise order may not have as much an impact; whereas chest muscles are not being utilized in other exercises.

Despite the lack of evidence showing exercise order may not have the impact we once thought it did for muscle growth for certain body parts such as arms and deltoids, keep in mind from earlier chapters that multi-joint exercises cause greater central fatigue than single-joint exercises. It is best from a fatigue perspective to keep the multi-joint exercises at the beginning instead of later in the workout. Also, keep in mind that an exercise like the squat will require more coordination than a leg extension. Your form is much more likely to deteriorate when leg extensions are performed first than after squats. Think about the amount of fatigue you get from squats and deadlifts instead of exercises like forearm curls or calf raises. You can do these all day with no tremendous impact on central nervous system fatigue because it's mostly peripheral-based fatigue. To maximize muscle growth, exercise order should emphasize the lagging muscles groups first in the workout when exercise motivation and energy are the highest. Exercise order has an impact on strength gains; therefore, exercises that are the most difficult to perform should be performed first.

---

475 Lucas Brandão et al., ~Varying the Order of Combinations of Single – and Multi-Joint Exercises Differentially Affects Resistance Training Adaptations,~ *Journal of Strength and Conditioning Research* 34, no. 5 (May 2020): 1254–63.

MUSCLEGATE: MULTI-JOINT MOVEMENTS ARE ALL THAT IS NEEDED

THE TRUTH EXPOSED: The advantage of compound movements like squats and bench press is that it correlates with increases in many muscle groups growth as opposed to isolation exercises, which increase individual muscle growth in specific areas. For example, the bench press can result in greater chest muscle activation, triceps, and anterior deltoids. In contrast, the dumbbell fly had much lesser muscle activation of these muscle groups, but greater activation of the biceps.[476] A 2017 study compared a multi-joint workout (bench press, squats, military press, etc.) to a single-joint exercise alternative workout (pec deck, leg extension, dumbbell lateral raise) with equal volume. At the end of the study, the multi-joint exercise group had better overall cardiovascular fitness. Muscle growth was also similar between groups; however; there was a greater trend for the multi-joint group to gain muscle while losing fat.[477] It's best to use a combination of both compound movements and isolation exercises for optimal muscle growth.

Some say all you need is multi-joint exercises and that isolation exercises are a waste of time. A 2017 review of the literature found that single-joint exercises were unnecessary to maximize size and were only beneficial for correcting muscle imbalances.[478] However, new research in the past five years has found that *single-joint exercises result in specific increases in muscle growth regions that differ from multi-joint exercises.* For example, one study compared triceps growth with:

---

476 Tom Erik Solstad et al., "A Comparison of Muscle Activation between Barbell Bench Press and Dumbbell Flyes in Resistance-Trained Males," *Journal of Sports Science & Medicine* 19, no. 4 (November 19, 2020): 645–51.

477 Antonio Paoli et al., "Resistance Training with Single vs. Multi-Joint Exercises at Equal Total Load Volume: Effects on Body Composition, Cardiorespiratory Fitness, and Muscle Strength," *Frontiers in Physiology* 8 (2017): 1105.

478 Paulo Gentil, James Fisher, and James Steele, "A Review of the Acute Effects and Long-Term Adaptations of Single – and Multi-Joint Exercises during Resistance Training," *Sports Medicine (Auckland, N.Z.)* 47, no. 5 (May 2017): 843–55.

- Bench press.

- Triceps extension.

- Triceps extension, then bench press, and

- Bench press, then triceps extension.

Triceps growth was +4.6% with just bench press, but bench press with triceps skull crushers resulted in an 11.5% increase in muscle growth in the triceps.[479] Another interesting observation was that the bench press was quite effective at stimulating the growth of the lateral head of the triceps, but other regions of the triceps, such as the long and medial head of the triceps, were not stimulated effectively. The group that trained with skull crushers had more growth of the lateral and medial heads of the triceps. This suggests that single-joint exercises cause regional muscle growth, not stimulated by multi-joint exercises alone. A 2021 study found that biceps growth was superior with a single-joint exercise than with a multi-joint exercise. In the study, subjects performed a supinated dumbbell row (multi-joint exercise) with one arm, and the other arm did biceps curls (single-joint exercise). Subjects performed 4-6 sets of 8-12 reps to failure of each exercise twice per week. If all you need is multi-joint exercise dogma was correct, then the dumbbell rows should have increased bicep growth because the bicep is heavily recruited during one-arm dumbbell rows. Bicep growth was nearly double in the bicep curl (11.1%) compared to the dumbbell row (5.2%).[480] Another study comparing a multi-joint exercise protocol alone to a combination of single and multi-joint exercises found that a combination of multi and single-joint exercises resulted in greater

---

479 Lucas Brandão et al., ~Varying the Order of Combinations of Single – and Multi-Joint Exercises Differentially Affects Resistance Training Adaptations,~ *Journal of Strength and Conditioning Research* 34, no. 5 (May 2020): 1254–63.

480 Pietro Mannarino et al., "Single-Joint Exercise Results in Higher Hypertrophy of Elbow Flexors Than Multijoint Exercise," *Journal of Strength and Conditioning Research* 35, no. 10 (October 1, 2021): 2677–81.

flexed arm measurement (4.39%) than multi-joint alone (3.50%).[481] You get more bang for your buck with compound joint exercises, but you still need to include single-joint exercises in your routine. If you are crunched for time, then choose the multi-joint exercises as a time saver. For optimal muscle growth, you need a combination of compound and isolation movement because each exercise stimulates muscle growth in different regions of the muscle.

MUSCLEGATE: THE HIP THRUST IS THE ONLY EXERCISE YOU NEED TO GROW THE GLUTES.

THE TRUTH EXPOSED: There has been an explosion of women doing hip thrusts; it's optimal for performing a wide variety of exercises to stimulate the glutes. The hip thrust mania came out of a research study where they hooked up electrodes to women's glutes and had them perform squats or hip thrusts. Hip thrusts resulted in greater glutes activation than the squat.[482,483] Game over, right? Well, not so fast. Just because a muscle group is activated more during exercise does not mean it's best for muscle growth. A 2020 study found increased glute growth when women trained with either the squat or the hip thrust; however, the squat resulted in greater glute growth. The squat increased glute growth by about 9.4%, and the hip thrust increased glute growth by 3.7%.[484] As mentioned earlier, it's best to do a combination of exercises for maximal muscle growth. As mentioned

---

481 Matheus Barbalho et al., "Influence of Adding Single-Joint Exercise to a Multijoint Resistance Training Program in Untrained Young Women," *Journal of Strength and Conditioning Research* 34, no. 8 (August 2020): 2214–19.

482 Walter Krause Neto et al., "Gluteus Maximus Activation during Common Strength and Hypertrophy Exercises: A Systematic Review," *Journal of Sports Science & Medicine* 19, no. 1 (March 2020): 195–203.

483 Jose Delgado et al., "Comparison Between Back Squat, Romanian Deadlift, and Barbell Hip Thrust for Leg and Hip Muscle Activities During Hip Extension," *Journal of Strength and Conditioning Research* 33, no. 10 (October 2019): 2595–2601.

484 Matheus Barbalho et al., "Back Squat vs. Hip Thrust Resistance-Training Programs in Well-Trained Women," *International Journal of Sports Medicine* 41, no. 5 (May 2020): 306–10.

earlier, performing a deep squat maximally activates the glutes during the squat. A meta-analysis concluded that the step-up exercise and its variations present the highest levels of glute activation, followed by several loaded exercises and its variations, such as deadlifts, hip thrusts, lunges, and squats.[485] Use a combination of step-ups, lunges, squats, and hip thrusts to maximize glute development. Finally, when you do squat, use a deep squat. Researchers compared glute growth with full squats below parallel to partial squat above parallel. Glute growth was greater for the full squat (6.7%) than the parallel partial squat (2.2%).[486] It can be suggested that the glutes are stretched more in a full range of motion compared to a partial squat. The hip thrust is a great exercise, but you need a combination of exercises for optimal glute growth.

CHAPTER SUMMARY:

- The muscle group you want to grow the most should be performed first.

- Start with multi-joint exercises first because they are the most fatiguing.

- Single joint exercises stimulate muscle growth in regions of the muscle that multi-joint exercises cannot.

---

485 Neto WK, Soares EG, Vieira TL, et al. Gluteus Maximus Activation during Common Strength and Hypertrophy Exercises: A Systematic Review. J Sports Sci Med. 2020;19(1):195-203.

486 Keitaro Kubo, Toshihiro Ikebukuro, and Hideaki Yata, "Effects of Squat Training with Different Depths on Lower Limb Muscle Volumes," *European Journal of Applied Physiology* 119, no. 9 (September 2019): 1933-42.

CHAPTER 17:

THE INTERFERENCE EFFECT

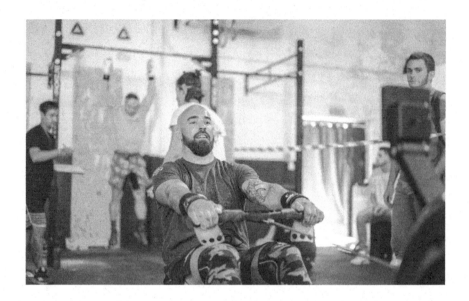

CARDIO AND MUSCLE GROWTH

It is common for lifters to perform cardio to enhance fat loss while increasing lean muscle mass. Over the past few years, several research studies have found that when cardio is performed back-to-back with resistance exercise, there seems to be a blunted muscle growth effect. This has led lifters to believe that they should not perform any cardio if attempting to gain muscle. The relationship between cardio and muscle growth is much more complex than people make it out to be. Aerobic exercise provides many beneficial effects on the cardiovascular system that cannot be achieved through resistance exercise; however, there are appropriate times to perform cardio that will not interfere with muscle gains.

MUSCLEGATE: CARDIO KILLS MUSCLE GROWTH GAINS

THE TRUTH EXPOSED: There has been a ton of research on this topic called the *interference effect*. The research has shown that performing cardio and weight training together can impair muscle growth. To be clear, cardio won't completely stop muscle growth gains, but it can slow down the process. Most research has been done on the leg muscles showing lower muscle growth when cardio and resistance exercise are combined. Some have speculated that it disrupts anabolic signaling pathways, glycogen depletion, excessive fatigue, etc.[487] Training with excessive aerobic exercise and resistance exercise results in fewer anabolic signaling pathways being stimulated. Cardio can take valuable resources (i.e., calories) away from muscle growth. Just like excessive volume with resistance exercise can have a negative impact on muscle growth, so does combining excessive cardio and resistance exercise. *The factors that determine whether combing cardio and resistance exercise together blunt muscle growth is the type of cardio you do, the volume and intensity of the cardio performed, and whether you do cardio in a close period with weight training.* High-intensity cardio after resistance exercise was found to result in less muscle growth (1.8%), whereas moderate-intensity exercise had a lesser effect (3.6%) compared to resistance exercise performed alone (4.1%).[488] One meta-analysis found that the greater the frequency and duration of cardio, the greater its impact on reducing muscle growth.[489] A 2021 meta-analysis found that concurrent training is more adverse seems for trained individuals compared to

---

487 Jackson J. Fyfe, David J. Bishop, and Nigel K. Stepto, "Interference between Concurrent Resistance and Endurance Exercise: Molecular Bases and the Role of Individual Training Variables," *Sports Medicine (Auckland, N.Z.)* 44, no. 6 (June 2014): 743–62.

488 Jackson J. Fyfe et al., "Endurance Training Intensity Does Not Mediate Interference to Maximal Lower-Body Strength Gain during Short-Term Concurrent Training," *Frontiers in Physiology* 7 (November 3, 2016): 487.

489 Kevin A. Murach and James R. Bagley, "Skeletal Muscle Hypertrophy with Concurrent Exercise Training: Contrary Evidence for an Interference Effect," *Sports Medicine* 46, no. 8 (August 2016): 1029–39.

untrained, but spacing your cardio apart from resistance exercise by three hours seemed to block the interference effect from reducing strength gains in trained athletes.[490]

Most studies looking at the interference effect have used running and weightlifting; *however, a recent meta-analysis found there is no impact of cycling and weightlifting on muscle growth.*[491] Researchers suspect that since running involves high eccentric contractions, like excessive eccentric training, this can cause excess muscle damage. Cycling does not have high eccentric contractions, hence less muscle damage. However, a recent study found that high-intensity cycling directly after resistance exercise can cause an interference effect for strength gains but not muscle hypertrophy. Researchers divided women into two groups. One group performed only resistance exercise for six weeks. The other group completed the resistance exercise and did high-intensity interval cycling 10 minutes after each lifting session. The cycling protocol consisted of 10 × 1-minute intervals at maximum aerobic power, with the workload being increased by 5% each week. There was 1-minute of passive rest between each interval. If you can imagine doing 10 one-minute maximal sprint sessions after a workout, you know how this study ended. The resistance-only training session had increases in power tests such as the countermovement jump, but the combined high intensity and cycling group did not. However, despite the differences in power production between the two groups, there was no difference in muscle size or strength between the two groups.[492]

---

490 Henrik Petré et al., ~Development of Maximal Dynamic Strength During Concurrent Resistance and Endurance Training in Untrained, Moderately Trained, and Trained Individuals: A Systematic Review and Meta-Analysis," *Sports Medicine (Auckland, N.Z.)* 51, no. 5 (May 2021): 991–1010.

491 Jacob M. Wilson et al., "Concurrent Training: A Meta-Analysis Examining Interference of Aerobic and Resistance Exercises," *Journal of Strength and Conditioning Research* 26, no. 8 (August 2012): 2293–2307.

492 Polyxeni Spiliopoulou et al., "Effect of Concurrent Power Training and High-Intensity Interval Cycling on Muscle Morphology and Performance," *Journal of Strength and Conditioning Research* 35, no. 9 (September 1, 2021): 2464–71.

If you must do cardio, make sure it is after resistance exercise. In a meta-analysis, researchers found that 1-RM was significantly less when resistance exercise was done before cardio.[493] If you perform cardio first, you can deplete valuable glycogen, which will lead to reduced subsequent resistance exercise performance and volume. Reduced glycogen stores have been found to negatively affect anabolic signaling pathways.[494] Combining both activities in a single session leads to greater glycogen depletion, increased sympathetic nervous activity, and increased stress hormones, impairing the recovery process.

Keep in mind that excessive cardio will result in a greater caloric deficit, and as you know, it's tough to gain muscle when you are in a caloric deficit. A recent meta-analysis found that an energy deficit impairs building muscle mass. They also found that an energy deficit of 500 calories per day prevented building lean mass in response to resistance training in a state of normal energy balance.[495] Most experts believe a caloric surplus of 300-500 calories per day can enhance lean muscle mass while minimizing unnecessary gains in fat. It is much easier to gain muscle if you eat a caloric surplus.

CARDIO IS NOT EVIL

Cardio should not be vilified. If done properly, you benefit from both without worrying about blunted increases in lean mass. Much of the research investigating the combination of cardio and resistance exercise performed together has found no impact on lean mass. A study that compared weightlifting alone to weightlifting plus cardio (i.e., separated by hours three

493 Zsolt Murlasits, Zsuzsanna Kneffel, and Lukman Thalib, "The Physiological Effects of Concurrent Strength and Endurance Training Sequence: A Systematic Review and Meta-Analysis," *Journal of Sports Sciences* 36, no. 11 (June 2018): 1212–19.

494 Andrew Creer et al., "Influence of Muscle Glycogen Availability on ERK1/2 and Akt Signaling after Resistance Exercise in Human Skeletal Muscle," *Journal of Applied Physiology* 99, no. 3 (September 1, 2005): 950–56.

495 Chaise Murphy and Karsten Koehler, "Energy Deficiency Impairs Resistance Training Gains in Lean Mass but Not Strength: A Meta-Analysis and Meta-Regression," *Scandinavian Journal of Medicine & Science in Sports*, October 8, 2021.

hours) found that only resistance exercise plus cardio had decreases in body fat (i.e., – 11%) compared to resistance training alone (i.e., – 6%). Both groups had similar increases in lean mass, but the combined cardio and weightlifting group had blunted peak power.[496] One crucial aspect of this study was that it controlled for calories, so that caloric needs were met with all groups, and each group received a whey protein isolate group post-exercise. Whether the interference effect is due to a blunted anabolic signaling pathway or results from being in a caloric deficit remains to be determined. There are several studies that have found that a combination of resistance exercise and cardio can result in decreases in body fat with increases in lean mass at the same time. [497,498]

Some lifters think they get all the cardio from weightlifting and doing high reps. One study had experienced weightlifters do squats and deadlifts to get their heart racing, whereas the other group did weightlifting and high-intensity aerobic exercise training. Both groups had improvements in cardiovascular function, but the strength training plus cardio group had greater cardiovascular improvements.[499] Many of the current strongmen that lift cars and atlas stones are now incorporating cardio (in the right dose) into their routines because it makes them overall better athletes. Cardio will result in

496 Matthew J.-C. Lee et al., "Order of Same-Day Concurrent Training Influences Some Indices of Power Development, but Not Strength, Lean Mass, or Aerobic Fitness in Healthy, Moderately-Active Men after 9 Weeks of Training," *PLOS ONE* 15, no. 5 (May 14, 2020): e0233134.

497 Shawn P. Glowacki et al., "Effects of Resistance, Endurance, and Concurrent Exercise on Training Outcomes in Men," *Medicine and Science in Sports and Exercise* 36, no. 12 (December 2004): 2119–27.

498 Brett A. Dolezal and Jeffrey A. Potteiger, "Concurrent Resistance and Endurance Training Influence Basal Metabolic Rate in Nondieting Individuals," *Journal of Applied Physiology* 85, no. 2 (August 1, 1998): 695–700.

499 Patroklos Androulakis-Korakakis et al., "Effects of Exercise Modality During Additional 'High-Intensity Interval Training' on Aerobic Fitness and Strength in Powerlifting and Strongman Athletes," *Journal of Strength and Conditioning Research* 32, no. 2 (February 2018): 450–57.

better muscle pumps by increasing the number of capillaries per muscle area, allowing more oxygen and blood flow to the muscle.[500]

Better blood flow to muscle with higher capillary densities can conceivably result in a better anabolic environment. This can be accomplished by low-intensity cardiovascular training.[501] One study *found that combined cardio and weightlifting may improve muscle growth.* The study investigated cardio in the morning with resistance exercise performed 6 hours in the evening or resistance exercise alone. The group that performed cardio and resistance training had greater increases in mTOR (i.e., increasing mTOR increases anabolic pathways) and increased VEGF (i.e., promotes new blood vessels). The author concluded that concurrent aerobic and resistance exercise *might enhance* muscle anabolic environment compared to creating a catabolic environment.[502] The key point is that this study separated cardio from resistance exercise by 6 hours; the studies that have combined them in one session have primarily resulted in adverse effects. If you do cardio with resistance exercise, make sure it is separated by 6 hours or preferably done on a different day. If you absolutely must do cardio and resistance exercise together, make sure the cardio sessions are short. Optimally, it is best to do cardio on opposite lifting days.

COMBATING THE INTERFERENCE EFFECT WITH NUTRITION

Most research on the interference effect has had subjects drink water during exercise. I suggest you drink 40 grams of whey protein and

---

500 B. J. McGuire and T. W. Secomb, "Estimation of Capillary Density in Human Skeletal Muscle Based on Maximal Oxygen Consumption Rates," *American Journal of Physiology. Heart and Circulatory Physiology* 285, no. 6 (December 2003): H2382-2391.

501 Naoko Shono et al., "Effects of Low Intensity Aerobic Training on Skeletal Muscle Capillary and Blood Lipoprotein Profiles," *Journal of Atherosclerosis and Thrombosis* 9, no. 1 (2002): 78–85.

502 Tommy R. Lundberg et al., "Aerobic Exercise Does Not Compromise Muscle Hypertrophy Response to Short-Term Resistance Training," *Journal of Applied Physiology (Bethesda, Md.: 1985)* 114, no. 1 (January 1, 2013): 81–89.

carbohydrate drink to replenish glycogen and increase protein synthesis during exercise and after exercise. The abundance of research shows that combined cardio and resistance exercise increases a protein called AMPK, which blocks anabolic actions in muscle. AMPK acts as a negative feedback loop on muscle growth by reducing muscle protein synthesis.[503] Still, AMPK is directly affected by nutrient availability (calories).[504] Whey protein and carbohydrates have both been found to increase AMPK levels and increase protein synthesis.[505] Maybe a cardio and resistance exercise protocol on an empty stomach senses results in low nutrient availability and depleted glycogen, which increases AMPK. Resistance exercise was thought to modestly deplete muscle glycogen, but we now know resistance exercise depletes much more glycogen than we previously thought. It has been estimated that an intense, high-volume bodybuilding style workout can *modestly* deplete glycogen anywhere from 24–40%.[506] A recent study had lifters perform a high-volume resistance exercise protocol. Total muscle glycogen decreased by 38%, but a different story arose when they analyzed the different muscle fibers. Type I fibers glycogen decreased by 33%, whereas, in type II fibers, there was a drop of 54%.[507] AMPK activity is

503 Rémi Mounier et al., ~Antagonistic Control of Muscle Cell Size by AMPK and MTORC1,~ *Cell Cycle (Georgetown, Tex.)* 10, no. 16 (August 15, 2011): 2640–46.

504 P. J. Atherton et al., "Selective Activation of AMPK-PGC-1alpha or PKB-TSC2-MTOR Signaling Can Explain Specific Adaptive Responses to Endurance or Resistance Training-like Electrical Muscle Stimulation," *FASEB Journal: Official Publication of the Federation of American Societies for Experimental Biology* 19, no. 7 (May 2005): 786–88.

505 Gabriel J. Wilson et al., "Leucine or Carbohydrate Supplementation Reduces AMPK and EEF2 Phosphorylation and Extends Postprandial Muscle Protein Synthesis in Rats," *American Journal of Physiology. Endocrinology and Metabolism* 301, no. 6 (December 2011): E1236-1242.

506 René Koopman et al., ~Intramyocellular Lipid and Glycogen Content Are Reduced Following Resistance Exercise in Untrained Healthy Males,~ *European Journal of Applied Physiology* 96, no. 5 (March 2006): 525–34.

507 Rune Hokken et al., "Subcellular Localization – and Fibre Type-Dependent Utilization of Muscle Glycogen during Heavy Resistance Exercise in Elite Power and Olympic Weightlifters," *Acta Physiologica (Oxford, England)* 231, no. 2 (February 2021): e13561.

regulated by glycogen availability.[508] Since low glycogen is associated with workout fatigue and reduced glycogen stores; it could help explain why combining excessive cardio and resistance exercise resulted in less muscle growth. If you are trying to put on muscle, it's probably best to limit cardio to low-intensity exercise. Low to moderate intensity cardio used as a recovery modality will enhance recuperation by increasing blood flow to muscle and improving cardiovascular health. I recommend limiting cardio to 25 minutes a week, preferably four times a week. This way, you are still getting the beneficial effects of cardiovascular training but maximizing resources to build muscle.

CHAPTER SUMMARY:

- Training with cardio and resistance exercise in excess can cause blunted muscle growth.

- The greater frequency, intensity, and duration of cardio, the greater its impact on reducing muscle growth.

- The interference effect seems to be more prominent with running, whereas cycling has less of an impact.

- Perform cardio preferably on the opposite day or if you have too spaced at least six hours away from resistance exercise.

- Cardio can improve cardiovascular function and improve blood flow to muscles.

- Cardio can enhance recuperation by increasing blood flow to muscle and improving cardiovascular health.

---

508 Natalie R. Janzen, Jamie Whitfield, and Nolan J. Hoffman, "Interactive Roles for AMPK and Glycogen from Cellular Energy Sensing to Exercise Metabolism," *International Journal of Molecular Sciences* 19, no. 11 (October 26, 2018): 3344.

CONCLUSION

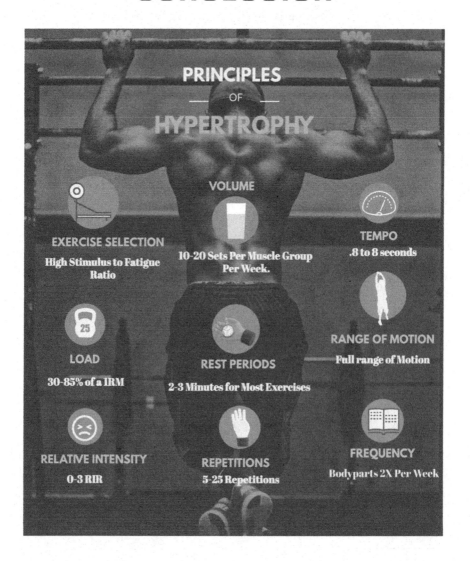

PRINCIPLES
— OF —
HYPERTROPHY

VOLUME
10-20 Sets Per Muscle Group Per Week.

EXERCISE SELECTION
High Stimulus to Fatigue Ratio

TEMPO
.8 to 8 seconds

LOAD
30-85% of a 1RM

REST PERIODS
2-3 Minutes for Most Exercises

RANGE OF MOTION
Full range of Motion

RELATIVE INTENSITY
0-3 RIR

REPETITIONS
5-25 Repetitions

FREQUENCY
Bodyparts 2X Per Week

Now that we have discussed the weight training aspect of muscle growth, it's also essential to discuss that it's critical to have the correct protein, fat, and carbohydrate ratios. Gaining muscle is always easier in a caloric surplus, but there is too much to cover and deserves a separate book.

GENERAL RECOMMENDATIONS FOR INCREASING MUSCLE

- Muscle growth can occur from a range from 30% to 85%.

- Using a combination of heavy, moderate, and light weight stimulates muscle growth while giving the joints and ligaments rest.

- Most of your reps should be performed a few reps away from failure (RIR of < 2).

- Only the last five reps with sufficient intensity are considered the ones capable of stimulating muscle growth.

- Perform each muscle group a minimum of 2–3 times per week.

- Increase volume when possible (minimum of 10 sets per week), depending on if you can recuperate from the previous workouts.

- Keep rest periods at 2–3 minutes or greater for larger muscle groups like the legs, chest, back, etc.

- Exercise repetition tempo should be from .8 to 8 seconds.

- Train the muscle groups you want to grow first in your workouts.

- Lighter loads (15–30 RM) can be used to stimulate muscle hypertrophy similar to heavy weight but should be taken close to failure.

- Using a heavier weight, training to complete failure is unnecessary.

- Repetitions should be completed thru a full range of motion.

- Time-saving training strategies: Drop-sets, rest-pause training, and supersets

- Consume a caloric surplus to gain muscle, with protein being .8-1.5 grams per pound of bodyweight spread over 4–6 meals per day.

- Prioritize sleep depending on individual preferences of 8-10 hours of sleep per night.

- Manage psychological stress in your life.

- Cardio can hinder muscle growth gains if performed in the same session; cardio should be performed on opposite days.

FURTHER
READING RESOURCES

The use of fitness misinformation has spread in recent years, leading to widespread consumer confusion on the real-world application of training and muscle growth. Many people are getting their training advice from Instagram and social media; however, very few reliable sources produce evidence-based bodybuilding information. There are several resources and books that I recommend for further reading and education for scientifically based articles on muscle growth and hypertrophy:

- MASS Research Review: https://www.strongerbyscience.com/mass/

- Weightology: https://weightology.net/

- Revive Stronger: https://revivestronger.com/

- JPS Health & Fitness: https://www.jpshealthandfitness.com.au/

- Chris Beardsley's Strength and Conditioning Research: https://sandcresearch.com/

- Stronger by Science: https://www.strongerbyscience.com/

- Renaissance Periodization: https://renaissanceperiodization.com/